CURING MY INCURABLE ECZEMA

CARA WARD

BOOKS BY CARA WARD

FICTION

Thirty-Minute Tales

WEIGHTING TO LIVE SERIES

Weighting to Live

Changes

Sixteen Months

Plus Uno

STANDALONE SHORT STORIES

Just Julia: A short story about eczema

Knock Down Ginger

NON-FICTION

Curing my Incurable Eczema

CONTENTS

AUTHOR'S NOTE

This is a graphic account of my battle with Topical Steroid Addiction which some readers might find distressing. All views expressed in this book are my own and provided for information purposes only.

This is not a manual on how to recover from eczema, Topical Steroid Addiction, or any other skin condition – it is simply an account of my own personal skin journey and a process I went through, and believed in, which resulted in me making a full recovery. I am not offering a magic pill and I definitely don't believe there are any quick fixes, and supplements/diet etc. can only help so much. What I went through was essentially a drug withdrawal – but more on that later …

I am not affiliated with ITSAN or any other official body and I am not a medical professional – I'm just a woman sharing her personal experience, and any information in this book is not intended as medical advice. For any medical advice, please seek help from a trained medical professional.

Some chapters and extracts have been taken from my blog, www.tswcara.blogspot.com, and the cover photo has not been touched up or filtered – the left half of the photo was taken nearly a month into withdrawal on 1st July 2013 and the right half was taken on 15th December 2017.

ANOTHER AUTHOR'S NOTE

Written 28th November 2022

Time is a funny one, isn't it, because just like our skin during withdrawal, so many things can change – like our views.

Since writing this book nearly five years ago, some of my opinions have changed, but instead of removing them, I've kept them in because it's how I felt at the time. Saying that, my views on withdrawal itself have remained the same – I'm a bit of a broken record in that regard.

I am pretty transparent about my views on certain subjects on my blog and Instagram account, so instead of elaborating in this book, I ask you to seek my opinions there x

To Mum
For there would be no book as I would never have been able
to get through withdrawal without you x

MONDAY 6TH MARCH 2017

This book has been a long time coming, and ever since I recovered from Topical Steroid Addiction back in August 2015, I have gone back and forth with the notion of writing a book about what I went through. In a way, it seemed like a no-brainer; I'm a writer and went through this incredible experience that completely changed my life and, as a result, I have a lot to say, but for some reason, I kept putting it off until it got to the point where a year and a half had passed and the book remained unwritten. In the last few months though I have thought more and more about it and have been 'itching' (sorry) to get the words down. Now, looking back, I think TSW is something that you need time to fully process, and I am finding it is only in the months since recovering that I have finally come to terms with it all. I needed space to reflect, to make sense of things, but now feels like the right time to put my story down in one place in order to move on.

At this point, I have no idea what I will say in the book, and my head is currently a mess of memories and feelings, but I find when I sit down to write, something takes over and I know exactly what to say.

Some facts and figures are hazy now as I never thought when I was going through withdrawal that one day I would be writing a book about my experience, but to my knowledge, everything I have shared with you is accurate.

As I mentioned in my author's note, this book is made up of new material along with posts and extracts taken from my blog, www.tswcara.blogspot.com, which I set up only a few months after recovering. Since then, it has become a friend and one of the most important things I've ever done, and knowing others have found it helpful, too, means the absolute world to me.

I hope you find this little book useful, and I am wishing you the best of luck on your journey.

Much love,
Cara x

P.S. All pictures of my journey can be found on my blog, www.tswcara.blogspot.com, or my Instagram, @carasnextchapter

WHAT IS TOPICAL STEROID WITHDRAWAL

his book is about a process called Topical Steroid Withdrawal that I went through to treat what I thought was eczema for many years, but was actually another condition called Topical Steroid Addiction.

I don't think even those of us who have gone through withdrawal know what it truly is. We can understand elements like the why – the reasons which led us all to make one giant, life-altering decision – but it's such a complicated and still largely ignored issue that I won't be going into much detail and will only be offering an overview of what I believe it to be. I am not a medical professional, I am simply a woman trying desperately to understand it all. One thing I do know for sure is that Topical Steroid Withdrawal is a totally needless process, but inevitably, for me at least, a necessary evil.

Topical Steroid Withdrawal (TSW) is essentially a drug withdrawal to 'cure' Topical Steroid Addiction (TSA). TSA is an iatrogenic condition, which simply means that it is brought on inadvertently by a medical treatment – in my case, topical steroids, although I believe that oral steroids (like Prednisone) also apply. It can sometimes be called Red Skin Syndrome (RSS) or Topical Steroid Withdrawal Syndrome (TSWS). I will be referring to it as Topical Steroid Addiction in this book, but, in my honest opinion, I don't believe that any of the names for our iatrogenic condition represent it well as they are either not inclusive (RSS) or exclude other forms of medication which can cause it (e.g. oral steroids).

This book is not intended to spread fear or panic so whatever you do, do <u>not</u> cease using any drugs without doing your own research, and please seek advice from a trained medical professional before embarking on something like TSW.

Not everyone who uses steroids will develop the condition. Through a lack of research, there is no clear reason as to why some develop TSA and others don't (I have my own personal theories which I won't be sharing as they are based only on a feeling).

Topical steroids in their varying potencies are widely used to treat skin conditions like eczema (which I initially had for about fifteen years) and for cosmetic use such as skin bleaching. Most require a prescription from a doctor, but there are some you can buy over the counter. They are available in different forms including ointments, creams, gels, oils and lotions.

I don't know where to start with the symptoms of TSA, but think of it as an exacerbated form of eczema (red burning skin, an intense bone-deep irritation and excessively dry, flaking skin unlike anything you have experienced before). These symptoms will more than likely appear after ceasing to use all steroids, which is why many think of it as eczema and not something else. That is what I thought for many years and countless doctors confirmed. The problem with steroids is that they work wonderfully for a period of time – a miracle cure – until they stop working, and to maintain your skin's condition, you need to use stronger and stronger steroids until they also stop working. The original eczema you used steroids for initially might have run its course, but you wouldn't know that as you now have this other condition which mimics symptoms, making it appear to be only getting worse, and spreading to areas you never had eczema in the first place.

When I first found out about Topical Steroid Addiction and the withdrawal process, I couldn't believe that I hadn't thought of it myself as it seemed so obvious – *of course* it was the steroids creating this mess my skin had somehow got itself into. I can safely say that I have never felt more sure of anything in my life, and I believed with all my heart that *this* was the answer I had been waiting many years to find. For me, this two-year gamble paid off and now I have better skin than I've ever had in my life. Going through TSW was the right decision for me and I believe for some of you reading this book, it will also be the right path, although it won't be easy, and over the next thirty or so chapters I will be sharing just how much of a toll it has taken on me physically and mentally, but how it's also picked up the pieces and put them back together again and along the way created a happier, healthier me.

There is still so much I don't understand, but one thing I do know is that TSW is life-changing.

MY ECZEMA HISTORY AND THE NIGHT THAT CHANGED MY LIFE

I suppose my skin story started when I was six months old when my mum noticed a tiny rash on my right wrist. Like any other parent would do, she took me to the doctor where I was very swiftly given the diagnosis that I had eczema, a condition as illusive and confusing as the treatment of it. I was prescribed hydrocortisone, a mild topical steroid cream, and soon that little patch blossomed and grew into something larger. Thanks to a mother who was naturally very cautious when it came to using any drugs, she applied them very sparingly and even though I did have eczema back then, it was never serious enough to impact my life – but I do believe that initial use of topical steroids when I was a baby turned the condition from a tiny patch into something much bigger. From about the age of seven my eczema wasn't a problem, until I went to secondary school. I am not going to go into that period of my life, but I will say that it was a very bad time for me; it shaped me, changed me from a happy child into a teenager who didn't like herself very much, and those changes showed in my skin with eczema rearing its ugly head. Now, when I look back, I would tell my young, teenage self that my eczema was probably caused by stress, but at the time, all I seemed to be told was that eczema was incurable and I had to find a way of 'managing' my condition which meant using emollients, moisturisers, steroids, immunosuppressants, bath preparations and lotions instead of looking for a reason *why* my eczema was coming up in the first place.

Apart from a nurse I spoke to in my teenage years called Jeanine who will forever be the best person I have talked to about my skin, I've been treated to a plethora of simply delightful doctors and dermatologists. Notable mentions go to the antiquated doctor (for some reason I remember he had a rather spectacular dent in his head) who looked directly at me, pointed his (in)experienced finger in my direction and told me, as if he was offering me words of profound wisdom, 'don't scratch'; or the doctors who would get their massive encyclopaedia of drugs and ailments out of a drawer to look for an appropriate cream, as if one size fits all. And last but not least, lest we forget, those who would be almost insistent upon me using steroids, immunosuppressants and the like before again reminding me that there is no cure for eczema.

I was fed this way of thinking for a very long time, and I believed it because you are conditioned to trust everything doctors tell you. I feel I need to say again that I am not blaming doctors and have immense respect for their profession, but in my lifetime, I have been treated by enough of them to feel justified to question the way in which eczema is treated by the medical community as a whole. You could tell me I'm wrong, but this is based on *my* experience and what I as an individual believe after having to go through the system for well over twenty years.

As a teenager my eczema was bad and at the time the only real treatments available to me were steroids, thick emollients, and all manner of fun stuff like that. It was around this time that I was referred to the hospital and started seeing dermatologists. I had skin tests which told me I was allergic to things that didn't make sense, and I remember a period where my skin was constantly infected and I had to keep taking antibiotics. I was seen by dermatologists at the hospital who would offer the same old treatments, but it wasn't until I was seen by a new dermatologist that things really went downhill. He was insistent I use steroids and would get angry if my skin hadn't improved. He was a big fan of Protopic, which at the time was being branded as a miracle cure, and his behaviour was so bad that it got to the point where my mum had to say to him that I was being bullied at school and didn't need to be bullied by a doctor as well. He did apologise for that, but things didn't change.

What happened next, I suspect, was the beginning of my addiction to steroids and the birth of Topical Steroid Addiction: I was prescribed (and ended up taking) a course of oral steroids which I am pretty certain was Prednisone. I was about fourteen at the time and as my poor immune system must have been pretty weak from all the drugs and antibiotics I had used, I really didn't stand a chance. Of course, we'll never know now what caused the condition to manifest and why – and I'm not here to name the doctors and dermatologists I've seen over the years as I think that is not going to help anyone (and it's certainly not what I want this book to be about).

Even as a teenager I knew steroids were bad and that if I continued to use the stronger creams I was prescribed I would only be asking for trouble, but at this point my skin was too bad not to use them so I tried to make the best of my situation and over time, gradually weaned myself down from Betnovate to Eumovate. After a while, I realised that for some reason, if I only put a bit of steroid cream on my hands and on a patch under my chin, it would control my whole body – I never touched the stuff as I hated the tingling sensation on my fingertips, so I would squeeze a pea-sized amount onto the back of my hand and use the back of both hands to rub it in. I would then swipe one of my steroid-covered hands over a small area under my chin. Even though I used Eumovate twice a day for years, it still felt like a better alternative to using something stronger. A few years before I began withdrawal, I was able to wean myself down to hydrocortisone 1%, applying it to the same areas. I thought maybe if I did it gradually, I might stand a chance of not having such a bad reaction when I stopped using them completely ... how wrong I was. This is why I don't believe in tapering.

I tried many times over the years to stop using steroids, each time hoping that perhaps my eczema would get better, but straight away, I'd get this awful reaction that I always assumed was my eczema coming back with a vengeance. I'd then book an appointment to see a doctor, but all they'd tell me was to use a stronger topical steroid or Protopic then throw in a new emollient for me to try. Even though I hated Protopic every time I used it, I was desperate to come off topical steroids, but it didn't take long for me to go back to them as I detested the side effects of Protopic, which for me included a painful burning each time I got in the shower or bath, a worrying increase in the amount of freckles I had even though I kept well out of the sun (I had to go to the hospital to get photos taken as there were so many), my face would flush red and the smell made me feel nauseous. Now, Protopic has been given a 'Black Box' warning because of its possible links to cancer.

Every time I went back to topical steroids, it was like reigniting a wonderfully familiar but toxic relationship – I knew it wasn't good for me, but my skin craved it. I had almost resigned myself to the fact that this was my life now and that steroid creams and immunosuppressants were always going to be a part of it. Over the years, along with other symptoms, I noticed my skin thinning badly, but I felt trapped – without these creams, my 'eczema' was only getting worse.

It wasn't until the summer of 2012 (a year before I started Topical Steroid Withdrawal) that things really started to change. Back when I had normal eczema and my skin wasn't addicted to steroids, my skin LOVED the sun, but now when it got hot, I would break out in hives and very strange rashes. As the UK never stays very hot for more than a few days at a time, my skin would calm down quickly, but when I went to Greece in July 2012, I found after a couple of days in the sun that my skin (especially on my legs and thighs) was coming up badly and I ended up spending the rest of the holiday covered up in the shade. I remember a few days before heading back to the UK when my supply of steroid cream was running dangerously low, frantically searching for it in Greek pharmacies, and when I was able to find some (I think it was Eumovate), I got back to my room and for the first time in years, literally slathered my entire body in it, desperate for the hives and rashes to die down. The cream did nothing though and it was only when I got back to the UK that my skin calmed down again.

For a few months, I was able to return to my normal routine of using hydrocortisone twice a day on the backs of my hands and under my chin, but over time, I found it increasingly hard to ignore just how thin my skin was. I wish I had taken photos as, especially on my face and the creases of my arms, you could see blue veins through my skin – it was really quite scary. I wore thick foundation which covered them, but it didn't stop the fear. But what could I do? I had severe eczema, which I was told was incurable, so had to find a way of 'managing' my condition.

In April 2013, I remember I was meant to sing at a friend's wedding which I was looking forward to, but had to cancel as an audition came up that could have been great for my career (at the time, I was making a rather half-hearted attempt at becoming a singer/actress) which I then had to cancel as the skin around my eyes suddenly swelled up really badly. Whilst all this was happening, I noticed a few rashes coming up on my arms and legs and I put hydrocortisone on the patches of 'eczema', but it had absolutely no effect. I went back to the doctors hoping they might have an answer, but all they suggested was to use the topical steroid Betnovate. My mum was also getting increasingly concerned about how thin my skin was. I think it was all coming to a bit of a head really and I remember feeling completely and utterly confused. At this point, I felt like I had two options:

1. Use stronger and stronger steroids until one day they would inevitably stop working or …
2. … I had no idea what my second option was, but knew I had to do something.

It wasn't until many weeks later on the evening of Thursday 6th June 2013 that I found an answer that would change my life forever. Earlier in the day, I remember my mum having a serious chat with me about how thin my skin was, but all I could say to her at the time was that I didn't know what to do as steroids were the only thing keeping my skin under control. Unable to shake off my mum's concerns though, I knew the time had finally come to sort out my skin once and for all so on a whim, that night, I typed into Google something along the lines of 'addicted to topical steroids' and instantly, I was given the answer I had waited over ten years to find – I didn't have eczema any more, but something called Topical Steroid Addiction. It was a total lightbulb moment, and I knew instantly that I would never use steroids again. That same evening, I started Topical Steroid Withdrawal and haven't looked back since. That was nearly five years ago now … and what a five years it has been.

I think what saved me in a way was going into

withdrawal blindly as I had no idea what was going to happen, but if I could sum it all up in one sentence, it would be to say that TSW was the best decision I have ever made for myself and my skin.

This book will document exactly what I went through during TSW – the good, the bad and the very, very ugly. This is not written by a medical professional with any kind of degree, but a woman who went through something life-changing. I am sharing my story in the hope that it can help others, but whatever I say, the decision of whether TSW is right for you must be yours and yours alone.

3

MY TOPICAL STEROID WITHDRAWAL

A lot of people have asked me over the last few years what my thoughts were before embarking on TSW, but I don't really have an answer as I went into withdrawal blindly having done next to no research with only the belief that I was doing the right thing. You see, I'm a terribly stubborn human and when I have made a decision, I tend to stick to it, sometimes with very little thought for the consequences.

I still feel emotional when I think of the moment I found out about Topical Steroid Addiction. It all seemed to click – *of course* my skin was addicted to steroids. I did my research as I went along which in a way, spared me from knowing what might happen next. Back in 2013 there were only a handful of blogs and people on the ITSAN forum documenting their journeys through withdrawal and even though I knew it was going to be hard, I certainly wasn't prepared for what happened next …

YEAR ONE
(Thursday 6th June 2013 – Thursday 5th June 2014)

Pretty much straight after I stopped using steroids, within a day or two, I got a rather lovely layer of golden crust above my top lip (I think they rather appropriately call it a 'crustache'). It freaked me out a little, but I found that if I gently flaked it off, I was able to cover the slightly sore skin underneath with moisturiser and foundation. During the first couple of weeks, my face was swollen and I was noticing my eyes becoming increasingly puffy, but with makeup, I was able to look relatively normal. Physically, I found even from the beginning I was so tired all the time, and I remember going to brunch with a group of friends, feeling completely out of it and not able to concentrate on what they were saying. It was a type of exhaustion that felt nothing like the kind you experience when you haven't had a lot of sleep – more that my body and mind had worn down like a used battery.

In some wild and foolish fantasy, I thought things would stay like that for a while – slightly swollen, a little itchy – but I'd be able to keep on living my life. A couple of weeks in though, things suddenly took a turn for the worse and on the evening of Thursday 20th June

2013, I woke up feeling extremely uncomfortable. It's hard, over four years later, trying to piece together exactly what it felt like, but I do remember extreme soreness, burning and irritation. In an attempt to calm my angry skin down, my mum fanned me in the middle of the night with a large book and rolled a glass bottle of water that had been in the fridge over my skin which felt amazing. The following day, my mum and I went out for a walk where I stroked a neighbour's dog and that night, I was very itchy and woke up the next day with extremely swollen skin on my face and puffy eyes. It's hard to know if the dog was the reason, or if it was going to happen anyway, but I think sometimes when you are flaring (or about to), known irritants can easily exacerbate the situation. Even though my mum supported my decision and wouldn't have made me do anything I didn't want to, she suggested, because she was scared, that I use a little bit of steroid cream just to take the edge off my symptoms. I knew wholeheartedly that using steroids again was out of the question and I think this terrible reaction almost made my resolve stronger as it showed just what they were capable of, so why would I want to use them again? It would only be waiting under the mask of steroids, untreated and waiting to strike. I knew I just had to keep going. Even though my mum was still nervous, she accepted my decision to stay on this uncertain path and bought an electric fan for me which was a life-saver. It was very hot in the UK around that time and I found that the heat, on top of the symptoms, was very hard to deal with. That weekend, things only got worse, and my mum was really scared, but after reading a lot of blogs and doing her own research, she realised that how I was feeling was just part of the process, and I think from then on, she was behind me all the way.

Even when things were so bad back then, I was determined to continue living like normal and was adamant I was going to keep working, but in the end, I had to cancel shifts as it was just too bad. If I lived closer to work, I might have been able to manage it for a little longer than I did, but with a two-hour journey to get there, it was just too much. On Monday 24th June (nearly three weeks in), I really started going downhill and the red was spreading from my face to my neck with patches appearing on my arms and hands – my eyes were also continuing to get even puffier.

On Friday 28th June, I went to bed just after midnight, but woke up a few hours later feeling extremely uncomfortable; over time, my sleeping pattern was becoming increasingly more fragmented. I got back to sleep after another few hours and the next morning, determined to keep living, I went to a shopping centre with my mum that was about an hour away. I was OK going there, but soon felt exhausted and so uncomfortable. My symptoms were also becoming increasingly harder to conceal – my face was very swollen and my eyes were so puffy that I felt like I had about eight eyelids. I remember taking my first photograph from withdrawal that day in a changing room and now, looking back, I wish I hadn't waited three weeks to document my journey as I would have been fascinated to see how my skin changed every day. I think it was at that point I realised work was going to be out of the question for a while and as my mum said she'd support me financially, I gave in to how I was feeling and accepted that I couldn't carry on as normal.

On the morning of 1st July, after having the best night's sleep since starting withdrawal, I felt so much better ... until I looked in the mirror and got the biggest shock of my life. My face had swollen to such a degree that it had completely distorted my face and my eyes were two puffy slits I could barely see through. The colour of my skin was also so red in places that it looked purple. I remember the skin on my face had wept through the night leaving a golden crust in its wake and I could only move my mouth a fraction. I recall hiding behind the door to the living room and warning my mum not to get a shock when I came in, but when she saw me, she couldn't help but suggest that she call a doctor and even though I wasn't sure I wanted her to, I agreed. Unfortunately (or maybe fortunately), the only doctor available that day was the one I saw just before starting withdrawal who suggested I use Betnovate so I knew that was going to be a pointless trip as I was determined I was going to do this and didn't want anything (or anyone) to stop me. I took an antihistamine and my mum bathed my eyelids and around my mouth with cotton pads soaked in warm water which meant I could eat, but it was still a struggle. By the afternoon, my skin had calmed down slightly, but I felt totally and utterly exhausted. The swelling in my face may have gone down a little, but my symptoms on the whole worsened.

Exactly a month into withdrawal on Saturday 6th July 2013, even though I couldn't work anymore because my symptoms were too bad, one of my close friends was having a birthday meal in London and I was determined to go. I remember on the morning of the lunch, my mum said whilst bathing my eyes that maybe I shouldn't go, but I was adamant that I was – I mean, I felt terrible, looked terrible and hadn't slept well in days, but I had one final shred of resolve that TSW wasn't going to interfere with my life spurring me on. I ended up going and I remember the further into my journey I went, the worse I felt, and I have a rather awful memory of a man sitting next to me on the tube who looked at my face then got up and moved as far away from me as possible. I am not condoning his behaviour, but I think that probably gives you an idea of how bad my symptoms were at the time. Looking back, I definitely shouldn't have gone. Whilst everyone was in pretty summer dresses and looked fabulous, I was in a plain tunic top which was the only thing I could stand wearing, and had three battery-operated fans on the table beside me to keep me cool. My friends were so supportive, and it was wonderful seeing them, but I felt so out of place being there and in reality, all I wanted to do was go home, take my tunic top off (as I couldn't stand wearing clothes for long periods of time), and proceed to sleep and scratch for the rest of eternity. That was the last time I saw my friends for over two years. After that, I decided to come off Facebook and pretty much became a hermit as (1) I wasn't well enough. (2) I really didn't want to think about what I was missing out on and (3) part of me felt like I needed some real time away from things to properly sort my life out.

During the first couple of months the red, swollen skin descended over my whole body, starting on my face and working its way south, and you can even see in photos the 'rash' spreading over time. The areas which got really irritated first were behind my knees and my back, but what's interesting is that they were also the first places to get better.

That summer, and those first few months of withdrawal, are now this rather weird blur, but I remember parts of it being truly horrific. I barely slept, I scratched (more like gouged at my skin) until I had created countless wounds, my skin burned – like someone had poured acid over me – and the entire top half of my body from my face to my lower back was weeping. I remember feeling at the beginning of withdrawal almost like a plate of jelly as certain parts of my body, especially my arms and lower back, were so swollen with unshed ooze that they would wobble as I walked. I would occasionally experience nerve pain which felt like little electric shocks, and the sensation of bugs crawling over my skin, and was pushed to a limit both physically and mentally that I didn't know I could reach. Over the first few months of withdrawal, the UK experienced a heatwave – one of the hottest summers in years – which only added to my discomfort. It's strange, but not once during that terrible time did I think about using steroids again and the worse it got, the more determined I became. I think I just knew I was doing the right thing and didn't want to see doctors – I didn't want to see anyone – I just wanted to get through it, which I knew I would eventually.

Even from the beginning, I sensed it was going to take a few years to fully recover, but I thought my symptoms would at least gradually get better over time and at some point, I'd be well enough to resume my life. My mum thought it would take six months, and my friends assumed I'd be back within a year, but to try and fathom how long this process will take, and second guess symptoms, is the most fruitless, pointless endeavour during withdrawal. Being realistic kept me from giving up. As time passed, the more friends would ask very subtly if I was doing the right thing. I would say yes and that would be that. Thankfully, after a few months, the weather cooled, my weeping subsided, and some of the swelling died down. I slept as much as possible (which wasn't a lot) and distracted myself by only watching positive things – anything negative I had to turn off immediately. I'd watch *Jonathan Creek* into the early hours and *Father Ted*, Graham Norton and Ellen DeGeneres if I needed to laugh.

The first six months of withdrawal were hell and even though the weeping subsided, the itch didn't let up one bit. I will elaborate on my symptoms in a later chapter, but looking back, I am amazed I was able to get through it. After that, even though my condition was still severe, I did start to notice small improvements and certain areas of my body, like my legs, were nearly back to normal. I thought at this point that I would have a gradual recovery, but just over a year in, I had an anniversary flare, which many experience through withdrawal. Thankfully, there was no oozing or oedema and I was finding that I was able to sleep more through the night, but that didn't mean it wasn't hard.

YEAR TWO
(Friday 6th June 2014 – Friday 5th June 2015)

After my anniversary flare, things generally calmed down and my symptoms became more isolated to my face, neck, hands and wrists (where I mostly applied topical steroids) with smaller patches on my arms and torso, but it was around this time that my left ankle suddenly, without warning, started flaring badly. I also continued to experience the feeling of burning on my skin with occasional nerve pain and the sensation of bugs crawling all over my body. To this day, I still don't understand why I had such trouble with my left ankle as I don't think I ever applied steroid cream anywhere near the area. My ankle started getting progressively worse during the second year until it was swollen, weeping and intensely itchy. There were times I couldn't wear shoes because of the swelling, and walking on it was too painful as the skin would just split. Even though my hands were bad during the first year, after my anniversary flare, they took a turn for the worse with symptoms very much like my ankle (swollen, bone-deep itching with wounds that wouldn't heal) and there were times where the fluid and swelling left me unable to move them much at all. My mum started having to wash my hair for me – do everything for me really – and I remember looking at my hands almost as if I was having an out-of-body experience. I obviously saw how bad they were, but I don't think I came to terms with the fact that they were *my* hands if that makes sense.

My face was still bad, but thankfully not like the symptoms I experienced on my hands, wrists and ankle and more of a vanity issue at this point. I found my face hard to deal with mentally as even though quite a lot of the swelling had gone down and was surprisingly not itchy in the slightest, I was left with this thick, rubbery skin which made me look a little more like my old self than I had done since starting withdrawal, but slightly distorted and I was worried this was now my new face. I was terrified that my skin was permanently damaged and the elephant skin was what I would have to deal with for the rest of my life. Back in 2014, not many people were talking about the elephant skin – they definitely documented the itching, the weeping and insomnia, but not this weird stage.

One more surprising guest star symptom which showed up uninvited to the party in the second year was excessive sweating. Like my ankle, it came out of nowhere and was definitely one of the worst things I experienced through withdrawal. After hearing about all my other symptoms, you would think a harmless bit of sweating would be a piece of cake … but imagine the feeling of saltwater going on an open wound (of which my body had plenty) and the feeling of being constantly damp. The other issue with it was that next to nothing could set it off – I'd just wake up drenched in it or I would talk on the phone and get slightly excited then start sweating. If it was just under my arms, it would have been OK, but this was a full body deluge of salty water.

I remember the second year of withdrawal as this long, stagnant phase tinged with doubt, discomfort and fear and from about eighteen months in, I really started to question whether I would ever make a full recovery. Looking back over photos I had taken from the beginning of withdrawal, it was obvious I had come a LONG way, but after feeling like I hadn't made any improvements for months on end, I was scared that this was it. I would then torture myself by looking at old photos pre-TSW and almost resigned myself to the fact that I would never look like that again. I always knew I was going to stick with TSW, but as time wore on, and I saw other people recovering quicker than me, I wondered if perhaps I was the one who just had 'incurable' eczema.

As time passed, and my recovery appeared to come to a halt, my positivity and determination trickled away. *Would I ever get better?* I remember in January 2015 (about twenty months in), I was meant to go to the theatre. Arrangements had been made to make my journey as comfortable as possible (including someone driving me there and back), but on the day, I was just too unwell. My skin was burning, I found it hard to wear clothes for any extended period of time, my left ankle was too swollen to stand on, the sweating was ridiculous, and I was desperately itchy and just too uncomfortable to leave the house. I cancelled the theatre trip with my friend and let doubt continue to creep in.

When spring arrived, my skin improved, but the changes were minor. I was able to start going out for short walks as my ankle was less swollen and the burning had also calmed down a little – I could even see small patches of white peeping through the red on my hands. I think around May 2015, I was so desperate to get out that my mum and I planned a trip to a town about forty-five minutes away by bus. I remember in the days leading up to it that I wanted to look nice so I straightened my hair for the first time since starting withdrawal, but the night before, my hands and ankle were so bad that I had to admit defeat as I knew I couldn't go. That made my doubt and fear resurface and I remember wondering if I would ever be able to return to real life again.

Summer arrived and with it brought more improvements. I was able to go out on longer walks as the burning had subsided and the sweating was getting better. My hands and ankle still weren't great though and there were days where they would weep and I would scratch until I felt like I was losing my mind. The elephant skin on my face was still an issue, but I think at this point I had just accepted that this was how I'd look from now on.

In mid-August (Monday 17th August 2015 to be exact), I looked in the mirror and saw a woman in the reflection that I hadn't seen for over two years. I looked at my hands – they were better, too, and so was my ankle, bar a little bit of redness. I feel like a total fraud saying all this but really, things did change so suddenly for me and it was as if one day I was going through withdrawal then the next, I wasn't. I didn't have this dancing for joy moment as, for a while at least, I don't think it sunk in that I was no longer in withdrawal … but slowly, as the months passed, happiness pushed its way through. I had recovered from Topical Steroid Withdrawal.

4

SYMPTOMS OF WITHDRAWAL

I have divided this chapter into two parts which will cover both the physical and mental symptoms. Topical Steroid Addiction is so much more than a skin condition and can easily take over your whole life – be your life. The physical symptoms are bad enough, but it's the mental ones that take the longest to recover from which can be overlooked in lieu of the physical. It's natural to feel anxious just as much as it is to scratch. I may have blanked out other symptoms I experienced through withdrawal, but I have tried to make this as detailed as possible which I hope will alleviate any fears you have as it's so easy to feel like you are the only one suffering.

~

• PHYSICAL SYMPTOMS •

OOZING/WEEPING SKIN

This was a symptom I experienced rather severely during the first three or so months of withdrawal. Practically the entire top half of my body wept – I'm talking my face, neck, arms, back and chest. It is one of the most unpleasant experiences and it's hard to put into words, but I remember this very subtle feeling just before my skin would start weeping, followed by a sinking in my chest as I knew what was coming next. I really found the sensation quite awful, as if you were draining – quite literally I suppose. I would pat the ooze away with tissues during the day and sleep on old pillowcases to try and soak it up overnight. I remember my lower back being particularly bad at one point and I would wake up to find these deep yellow patches on the sheets where my skin had wept. I always dreaded scratching back then as I knew it was only going to make my skin ooze more – which it did rather spectacularly. I am so grateful that the weeping didn't last on such a grand scale like that as it can really bring you down and sap you of what little energy you have left. As time passed, the weeping became more localised to my hands, wrists and left ankle until it stopped completely and hasn't returned since.

OEDEMA/SWOLLEN SKIN

This was something that went gradually over time, but like most of the more extreme symptoms, was more prevalent during the first six months of withdrawal. It's very hard to explain, but my skin towards the beginning of TSW almost felt as if it was made of some kind of thick jelly. I remember my arms and the 'muffin top' area of my torso especially being extremely swollen and weighed down with fluid. There were times where my skin felt uncomfortably tight and stretched and when it was like that, what I found helpful was to massage the area which would bring down the swelling a little.

For a long time, the lower part of my face was quite swollen, distorting my features, and I think after a while, you grow so used to this new person that you almost think it's how you will look for the rest of your life, but like every other symptom, it goes eventually.

PUFFY EYES

This is a symptom that started at the beginning of withdrawal and only got worse over the following few months, and to this day, it baffles me that I don't have any loose skin around my eyes. For many months, my eyelids were swollen and in the first three months, they would also weep. This was a symptom that gradually got better over time, and to anyone who is frightened that their skin might not recover, it will. Just give it time.

BONE-DEEP ITCHING

The itching through Topical Steroid Withdrawal was unlike anything I'd ever experienced in my life. They call it a bone-deep itch as it feels like the irritation is nestled deep within your body and for me at least it was a constant throughout the entirety of my withdrawal. This still baffles me but for some reason, my face never felt itchy – even at the beginning when it was weeping and swollen. I did notice that the way most areas of my body recovered corresponded to where I scratched the most first. I remember at the beginning of withdrawal, the worst places were my back and behind my knees, but they were also the first areas to get better. Then my hands, left ankle and neck, which were the last places to get really irritated were also the last to recover.

I tried to stop myself from scratching, and I remember nights where I'd tape cotton gloves to my hands, but they would inevitably be flung off after approximately five seconds so I could scratch again. I found that nothing really helped when my skin was very irritated, but there were times where I was able to find some relief by rolling a glass bottle filled with cold water over my skin which would sometimes be enough to stop myself from scratching. Looking back over it all with everything I know now, I do believe, within reason, that we are *meant* to scratch – it's as if the body wants us to be rid of this bad skin and by scratching it off, we are doing just that. This is in no way an invitation to rip your skin open with wild abandon, but more a plea to not feel bad for doing something that would be impossible not to do. I feel it is about time for my chapterly reminder that I'm not a doctor and this is only my opinion and not intended as medical advice.

I have heard that a lot of people going through withdrawal use artificial nails to stop the skin from tearing, but as I never tried them, I cannot offer any advice in that department. My attempt at trying to minimise the damage from scratching was to use a round-toothed comb as the teeth were blunt enough to not break open the skin … but if I'm being perfectly honest, it wasn't a great solution and most of the time, it wouldn't get to the itch so I'd have to resort to using my nails.

Another implement of sorts which I used to scratch my skin – that I would NEVER recommend but got immense relief from – was one of those high street loyalty cards. I cannot tell you how bad it was for my skin, but at that point, I was desperate. As I had cut my nails down to the lowest point physically possible, this card seemed to be the next best option. Bless my poor mum; in a bid to keep my skin from getting infected, she would wash this damn loyalty card twice a day to keep it clean as she knew I wasn't giving it up. After a while though, I just had to stop using it as it really caused a lot of damage, and I remember calling up the company the loyalty card came from and saying I had lost it and needed a new one ...

When I was in a scratching S.O.S. situation where nothing would hit the irritation, I would beg and plead with my mum to scratch me as she has, hands down, the best scratching nails known to man. She obviously hated doing it, but in the end, she wanted me to have some relief and it is only now, looking back, that I realise what a terrible position I put her in.

Apart from the inevitable cracked, open skin, some of the other side effects I experienced from scratching were infected puss-filled nail beds and cuticles, nails which dipped in the middle from being worn down and bruising from the intensity of my scratching.

DRY SKIN/SHEDDING

I think it's safe to say that none of us going through withdrawal have ever seen dry skin and shedding like it. You go through this cycle of flaring, weeping and redness followed very quickly by dry, flaky skin that is so extreme, there is a constant need to hoover and brush down anywhere you have been. For the first six months, the flakes were large and really gritty and there were times where there was so much dry skin after sleeping that my bed felt like a sandpit. I would wake up in the night and feel it all around me and have to brush it off completely otherwise it would be too uncomfortable, and anywhere I sat would soon be covered in skin. As time wore on, the flakes got smaller and softer, but it took the full two years for it to go completely.

I still find it novel that I can wear black now and not have to worry, and times where I'll look at the bed thinking I need to brush it down before remembering that I don't have to anymore. By the end of withdrawal, I was amazed I had any skin left and couldn't believe how lovely it was. Skin is the most incredible organ and I find it fascinating how it is able to rid itself of the skin it doesn't want any more then regenerate.

CRUSTY SKIN

This was the first real symptom of TSW that I experienced. I remember waking up a day or two after starting withdrawal with this thin layer of golden crust above my top lip, which is rather appropriately called a 'crustache'. I was able to flake it off and cover the slightly sore skin underneath with make-up and after a few days, it vanished. As time wore on, a thick crust would form wherever the skin had been weeping and in my (non-medical) opinion, I would just leave it alone – trust me, as someone who has suffered quite severely from the skin picking disorder Dermatillomania in the past, I know how tempting it can be, but picking it off is not a good idea. The crusty skin will come off when it's meant to.

CRACKS IN THE SKIN

Through withdrawal, I had cracks and open wounds all over my skin, and not just small ones, but deep, painful cuts. Some no doubt occurred because of the incessant scratching, but other times, the skin would just split open with very little provocation and I remember having some nasty looking lesions on my neck, arms, hands, lips and face. I was lucky and somehow none of them ever got infected, but that is something you've got to be aware of so please seek help from a trained medical professional if you suspect you might have an infection.

RED SKIN

My skin was most certainly red through withdrawal. For me, it started on my face before trickling down my body, and in my photos, you can actually see the redness descending – and we are not talking about slightly red here, but an angry, swollen, *burning* red. I remember one of my mum's friends who came over when I was maybe a month or two into withdrawal said I looked like I had been in a fire. By the second month, I was pretty much a tomato, but what I found fascinating, like most people, is that you are left with these white palms and a line on your wrists where the redness begins (they call it a red sleeve) – and let us not forget the reverse Rudolph white nose you will more than likely experience. Over time I found that the redness calmed down on its own and the only thing that helped was to keep cool. To take some of the anger out of my skin, I would sometimes roll a glass bottle filled with cold water over it. Some also suggest using ice packs, but I think I'd find that *too* cold if that makes sense. Like everything to do with TSW, I believe my good old friend time is the only true 'healer'.

*Please note, I am Caucasian, and red skin of course depends on ethnicity. On darker skin tones, the colour may become darker and change during withdrawal. We are all beautifully different x

BURNING SKIN

For me, this was one of the most debilitating symptoms of withdrawal, especially when I went out (which was rarely). Ranging in intensity, it almost felt like someone had poured acid over my skin. When I *did* go out, even if the weather was mild, I found that my skin would start to burn – and this only let up a few months before making a full recovery.

I remember all I wanted to do through withdrawal was go out, wear nice clothes and feel comfortable again so now being able to do that feels like such a luxury and it's something I know I will appreciate for the rest of my life. The only thing I found that helped was to keep cool and wear as little as possible to give the skin space to breathe.

NERVE PAIN

Thankfully, for me at least, I only experienced this symptom occasionally. You get these awful nerve zaps all over your body – think of it like little electric shocks – that can range from mild to severe. It's not pleasant, and the only thing I could do really was just wait it out and distract myself until it calmed down again.

THE FEELING OF BUGS CRAWLING ALL OVER MY BODY

Like the nerve pain, I luckily didn't experience this on a regular basis, but nevertheless, it definitely still had an impact on my withdrawal. Usually accompanied by the nerve pain, it was like having thousands of bugs crawling all over my body – so much so that at times I had to check there weren't actually bugs on my skin. It's disconcerting, uncomfortable and scary and I remember one time only a few months in when I was in the middle of a very nasty flare and it happened that it got to such an intensity that I burst into tears. I cried very few times during withdrawal – I can only remember three occasions – so it must have been bad.

Since recovering, I have experienced it very rarely – maybe every three months – and it will last for an hour or two before going again. It doesn't bother me much – just a mild discomfort – and there is no evidence of it on my skin; just the body trying to repair itself after years of damage from using topical steroids.

INSOMNIA

It's pretty much safe to say that for the first year of withdrawal I didn't sleep much at all and only then, it was in one to two-hour bursts. My sleeping patterns became so erratic that I'd take whatever I could get, having to resort to little sleeps during the day in an attempt to catch up. I hated going to bed at night and there were times where I'd sit on the edge of the mattress, scared to get in. The evenings only seemed to exacerbate symptoms, and nothing felt worse than waking up in the middle of the night to the feeling of gritty, dry skin in the bed all around me and having to desperately scratch or peel my skin off fabric which had wept into the sheets. Even though I was able to sleep for a few hours through the day, it always made me feel worse, and I think if I'd been able to sleep better during the night, that first year would have been so much easier to deal with.

You are probably wondering why, if I was so desperate to sleep, did I not just take sleeping tablets, but to be perfectly honest, my feeling at the time was that I was already going through a drug withdrawal and didn't want to replace those drugs with something else – I wanted to give my system a chance to recover naturally, without drugs. This might have been the wrong thing to do, and may have even prolonged my withdrawal, but it was what felt right for me at the time, and I think with something like TSW, you've got to listen to your gut instinct. I cannot tell you the difference it made in the second year when I started to sleep through the night – I mean, there were still times where I'd wake up once or twice, but on the whole, it was so much better and the difference it made was incredible as I was pretty much a zombie for the first year.

HAIR LOSS

I lost quite a significant amount of the hair on my head and eyebrows through withdrawal and had practically next to no body hair. Oddly, I didn't realise just how much I'd lost until it started growing back and now, looking at photos of myself from that time, my hairline was so set back it was scary.

I assume the hair loss was down to the extreme stress my body was under and in that case, I'm not surprised so much fell out. Amazingly, my hair and eyebrows are actually thicker now than they ever were before withdrawal and it's like nothing happened.

ELEPHANT SKIN

It is hard to know when this symptom began, but I can safely say that it became more prevalent in the second year. It also marked the start of a long, stagnant phase for me. Elephant skin is named for the thick, wrinkly skin you seem to get through withdrawal. Like with the swelling, it distorted my features and made me look a little more like my old self than I had done, but also different, which tricked me into thinking that this was what I would look like for the rest of my life. As the redness was much calmer in the second year – bar the places where I was flaring badly like my hands, left ankle and occasionally, my face – I really did despair that this was my new skin, but as this chapter suggests, it is a **symptom** of TSW, nothing more, and does go eventually. So many people have asked me what they can do for the elephant skin, but like everything else to do with TSW, all I can really say is to give it time.

Since recovering, it hasn't made an appearance and now my skin is completely back to normal. There have been times over the last two years where I have started to get really anxious and checked for signs of elephant skin, but there has been nothing. Always remember that the skin is capable of such incredible healing.

SWEATING

In the second year, after pretty much not sweating at all during the first twelve months, it was as if someone had turned on a rusty old tap and suddenly, I was drenched. I remember waking up covered in salty perspiration (even now, after everything I have told you, I really hate using the word 'sweat'). If I talked on the phone and laughed or got excited, I'd end up sweating – literally, the smallest thing would set it off. It was not just from under my arms either, but my whole body. I had to keep tissues near me at all times like I did with the weeping to soak it up and occasionally had to change my clothes (let's be real, my 100% cotton pyjamas) more than once over the day, but most of the time, it was so uncomfortable that I didn't even bother wearing anything on my top half at all. It also didn't help with the burning, and when sweat hit irritated or broken skin, it was hell. I've heard from many different sources now that sweating is a sign of healing, and I couldn't agree more. At some point during the second year, I started using a sensitive Mitchum roll-on deodorant, which obviously didn't help the rest of me, but definitely controlled the sweating under my arms. It took the whole of the second year to really sort itself out and now I sweat normally. Like most symptoms, just give it time.

A STRANGE SMELL ON MY SKIN

My mum remembers this vividly as during withdrawal, there was a very strange smell on my skin – she thinks it was like some kind of chemical whereas I remember it being a little more metallic. My mum said she would hug me sometimes and emanating from my scalp would be this sharp odour she'd never smelt before. I remember sometimes when I'd get in the bath, and my skin would hit the water, this smell would rise from the steam which I found mentally to be a bit of a blow. Even in the two years after recovering where I would have an anxiety attack and start to panic that I was going to flare, I'd smell my arms – just like I did back then – to check for *that* smell. It's never come back, but it will always stay with me, and my mum.

DRY/ITCHY/FLAKY SCALP

Thankfully, this lasted only a relatively short period of time. I think it was early on in the second year when my scalp started to get extremely dry and irritated and would weep occasionally. A few years before withdrawal, I remember using Head & Shoulders which really helped when I had bad dandruff, so I tried it again and couldn't believe how good it was with all TSA symptoms on my scalp clearing up extremely quickly. I used a sensitive 2-in-1 shampoo/conditioner and I don't know what's in the stuff, but it's brilliant, and I've heard of others going through withdrawal who swear by it, too. I still use the original shampoo as I absolutely love the brand.

I find it very interesting that in the years leading up to TSW, I had pretty terrible dandruff, but since recovering, for the first time in years, the natural oils have returned to my scalp and now, my hair actually gets greasy. You wouldn't think someone could get so excited by a greasy scalp, but to me, it's a very big deal.

SHIVERING

During the first year especially, even when it was warm, I remember shivering a lot and being very sensitive to the cold. There were times when I was so shivery that in a bid to get any kind of comfort, I'd have to stand over an electric fan heater just to try and feel warm again. It was so bad for my skin, but I was desperate as I hated the feeling of any clothes or layers on me. My body temperature regulated over time until it was back to normal and I haven't experienced any issues since.

• MENTAL SYMPTOMS •

DOUBT, FEAR AND WORRY THAT I'D NEVER GET BETTER

Due to the nature of our condition, and a shocking lack of research, we have very little medically to go on and most importantly, no crystal ball telling us *when* we're going to get better. As a result, teamed with the knowledge that it can sometimes take years to recover from, over time we are left with an almost constant sense of fear and worry that we might never get better. When I first heard about TSA, I had a lightbulb moment and knew instantly that this was the answer I had been waiting years to find, but as time wore on, I started to doubt whether I was doing the right thing. On top of all that, you've got to deal with countless doctors and organisations you are conditioned to trust telling you that there is no such thing as Topical Steroid Addiction – then, to make matters even worse, you'll look at your skin after months of flaring and pain and only see symptoms worsening. I think it's safe to say that it would take a person cast of solid stone to not let doubt and fear in. All I had to go on was a handful of blogs (with very few of them actually written by people who had recovered), a couple of doctors WORLDWIDE saying you would get better and my own personal beliefs.

For well over a year and a half of withdrawal I was pretty adamant that I would get better, but at around eighteen months in, I found myself questioning everything. It was a very dark time for me, but even in my most desperate of moments, I would never have gone back to using steroids or immunosuppressants again as I knew TSA would only be waiting for me when I stopped using them. Besides, they had *created* all these horrible symptoms in the first place. More than anything, I hope TSA is recognised so those suffering don't have to experience the doubt which can be crippling.

FEAR THAT I JUST HAD ECZEMA

This goes hand in hand with feelings of doubt and fear, but in the moments where I questioned if I was doing the wrong thing, I'd also wonder whether I was the one person going through withdrawal that just had 'incurable' eczema, but I think if you are on this path, rationally you know what you have now isn't eczema.

A SUDDEN, SEVERE PHOBIA

A few months into withdrawal, I developed a rather sudden and severe phobia of something that I won't share the name of just in case others are as affected by it as I was. Even the thought of this *thing* would send me into such a scratching frenzy that it nearly drove me insane. I'd never experienced anything like it in my life – it was just awful. The fear of it was so concentrated at one point that I was terrified I'd have it for the rest of my life, but as time passed, the phobia was gradually not there anymore and now, even though the *thing* in question is still something rather unpleasant, it doesn't affect me at all. So very strange.

ANXIETY

It's odd, but my anxiety only showed what it was capable of *after* I had recovered from Topical Steroid Addiction and through withdrawal, it was this other beast entirely. My anxiety manifested itself through TSW by heightening all my emotions like fear, doubt and worry then multiplying them in my mind until I'd worked myself up into such a state, I'd be paralysed by it. I think my anxiety was definitely responsible for the phobia I developed during the first year – an amalgam of emotions making my senses and vulnerable mind more susceptible to anything negative.

A DEEP SADNESS THAT I WAS MISSING OUT ON LIFE

I am going to be sharing an article I posted on my blog about this in more detail, but there were moments during withdrawal where I'd look at others my age living life and feel desperately sad that I couldn't do the same – even being able to do simple things like wearing nice clothes and going shopping. I deactivated my Facebook account through withdrawal as I didn't want to see what I was missing out on. TSW can make you feel like you are throwing your life away when in reality, it is *giving* you a life. I spent years using a drug that was slowly doing a lot of damage to my skin and body, but on reflection, TSW turned out to be the best thing I have ever done for myself and my skin.

POSITIVITY

After all the negatives, I thought it might be nice to end on a positive note. I will be writing an entire chapter on the subject as positivity played a massive part in my withdrawal, and even though I *did* suffer rather badly mentally, overall, the experience for me was a generally positive one where I learned so much about myself and completely changed as a person. After withdrawal, I found that the small things were the most precious and I even started to love myself … although that is still a work in progress. Sometimes, it's the things on the surface which appear to be bad that have the potential of being the most wonderful blessings.

• THE SYMPTOMS I HAVE EXPERIENCED SINCE RECOVERING •

ANXIETY, PANIC ATTACKS AND PTSD

Even though I experienced terrible symptoms mentally through withdrawal, it was only after TSW that these symptoms really showed their true colours. Don't get me wrong, it was very bad whilst I was going through withdrawal – especially when the doubt and fear really kicked in that I was doing the wrong thing – but nothing compared to the anxiety I experienced *after* TSW. I think it all stemmed from a rather acute fear of flaring again so when I'd see anything that could even remotely mean that might happen – like a minor rash – my thoughts would spiral out of control. To try and put my mind at ease, I'd start to over-analyse my appearance and feel for signs of elephant skin, or smell my arms for that strange chemical smell, but all it did was fuel the fires of anxiety.

There were times where it would reach such a head that I would actually start to see symptoms that weren't there and when it was very bad, I'd have a panic attack. If you have experienced them before then you will know just how terrible they can be – you almost feel like you are dying. I found during a typical panic attack that my throat would dry up, my heart would start pounding and my brain would almost feel like it was pulsing and too tight for my skull. Your mind becomes a blur of emotions and the thoughts that run through your head can be very dark indeed. It wasn't until well after a year post-TSW when I realised that I might have some form of PTSD, which a therapist confirmed, and has taken me a long time to come to terms with.

I sometimes get a little anxious (although nothing to do with TSW) and I'm still working on my confidence. There are times in social situations where I just want to be on my own and I think that stems from over two years of isolation through TSW. I will feel out of place like I'm behind and can't catch up, but then I'll remember that I went through something that changed me as a person for the better; grounded me, gave me the tools to see things from another perspective. That is what illness teaches you – it gives you a true understanding of what is important and that certainly isn't possessions; it's the small things and the people around you.

I am choosing to be totally honest about how bad the mental symptoms can get as I don't see the point of glossing over anything. TSW is just as hard mentally as it is physically and the goal of this book is to be totally transparent with you all about what can happen before, during and *after* withdrawal.

RASHES

I will occasionally get the odd minor rash that is simply that; a minor rash. They never develop into anything serious and after only a few days (if that), they will dry up and disappear. I would gladly take those rashes for the rest of my life if they are anything like the ones I have experienced since recovering. Back when I had eczema, I was told to keep my skin moisturised, and I always remember thinking it odd that moisturisers would only make rashes etc. worse and prolong any issue, as opposed to just leaving them to get better on their own. I would suggest down the line leaving all rashes alone – not putting moisturiser or anything on them – just to see what happens.

Even though the rashes I have experienced since recovering have been harmless, there have been times where they have made my anxiety go into overdrive – I'd see a rash, but in my mind, I was flaring. Try not to let anxiety get the better of you.

HAND FLARES

During the first year post-TSW from approximately October 2015 to summer 2016, I had various rashes and two isolated flare-ups on my hands. Those flare-ups happened both times I went to Verbier in Switzerland on work trips. It's hard to know what caused them to flare, but I think it was probably something to do with the altitude mixed with stress. Even though my hands were bad while I was there, it didn't affect my life and the difference this time was that the flares only lasted a handful of days as opposed to the sometimes months during withdrawal.

I have said this before, but I believe my hands were a year behind the rest of me in recovering as symptoms only really kicked in after a year into withdrawal. I also used steroid cream on my hands for well over ten years cumulatively and even though it seems like three years of pain is a big price to pay, I would go through it all again if it meant I had the skin on my hands that I do now. Sometimes the best things in life are those that were the hardest battles to fight.

DRY LIPS

Since recovering, my lips will occasionally get dry and chapped which I've now realised only happens when I have cold/flu symptoms or if my sugar intake has been higher over a period of time. Not really an issue though, and a bit of petroleum jelly once in a while works wonders.

NATURAL OILS

I suppose this isn't a symptom per se, but I felt like I had to talk about it in this chapter as it's something that's happened as a result of going through withdrawal. As you will probably know by now, I stopped using moisturiser and since recovering, I've noticed that the natural oils have been returning to my skin. There have been occasions where I have actually *seen* the oils on my face and gotten the odd spot because my skin is trying to find the right balance. One time during the winter of 2016, the skin on my back felt like it had been moisturised with a thick, luxurious cream, and even more crazy is that after what can only be described pre-TSW as the Sahara Desert on my scalp, it has actually been greasy which to me is a miracle! My skin takes care of itself now and I only use moisturiser on my legs to replace the moisture lost when I use shaving foam or dry body brush.

NERVE PAIN AND THE FEELING OF BUGS CRAWLING OVER MY SKIN

I mentioned this symptom earlier in the chapter where maybe every three months, for an hour or two, I will experience nerve pain (which feels like tiny electric shocks) and the sensation of thousands of bugs crawling over my skin. Weirdly, even though it's a little uncomfortable, I find it strangely comforting as I know it's only my body repairing itself – besides, nothing shows on my skin whatsoever; it's just a feeling.

SKIN BURNING

This is a symptom unlike the burning I experienced through withdrawal – more like a heat trying desperately to escape from my skin. It's not painful like it was during TSW – more disconcerting and actually, quite nice. It happens every few months or so – always at night and only lasts the evening. What's odd about it is my skin always looks incredible the next day. I would love to know what it is … then bottle it.

HIVES

From the summer of 2016 for over a year, I'd get occasionally get hives. There are reports out there which suggest they are one of the last symptoms of withdrawal and from my own personal experience, I'm inclined to agree. That summer, there was a period over a few weeks where I got a bout of hives on my chest, torso and back along with a strange rash which you couldn't really see, but my anxiety most certainly knew was there. I hadn't experienced any issues on those areas of my body for a long time – even during withdrawal – so it did make me nervous. At this point, I was also under a lot of stress and had a very bad cold with acute sinusitis so I am not sure whether it was down to illness, stress or just plain old TSW, but now, I think it was a mixture of all three. The hives and rash cleared up a few weeks later and I haven't experienced any problems in those areas since. Later in the year, I also got some hives on my hands which only lasted a few days and haven't returned.

I found that antihistamines helped a little, but to be perfectly honest, the best and only real advice I can offer you (...yet again) is to leave it all alone and let time take care of the rest.

Going into this chapter, I wasn't expecting it to be as large as it turned out to be and I have to say, writing it brought a lot back. Each symptom on its own is hard, so when you have to experience many together, it can be nothing short of unbearable. There have been cases where people can feel suicidal through TSW so if you ever feel like that, please seek help from a trained medical professional or call a national helpline immediately. You are <u>not</u> alone.

5

YOUR TSW SURVIVAL KIT

*T*his chapter is dedicated to the things I couldn't have lived without through withdrawal. I will not be including any dietary advice or suggestions on what drugs to take as we are all so different. Besides, I am not a nutritionist or medical professional.

COTTON PYJAMAS

These were pretty much the only thing my skin could tolerate through withdrawal. I got mine from Marks & Spencer as they didn't cling to my skin, were very comfortable and helped keep me cool. They also took a lot of abuse – whether it was from moisturisers, petroleum jelly, ooze or scratching – and lasted a long time, but were cheap enough to replace when I needed to.

COTTON CLOTHES

If you have to go out or need to work, invest in clothes that are 100% cotton as pretty much any other fabric is probably going to irritate your skin.

THIN, NON-WIRED BRAS

Ladies, trust me when I say that a nylon, underwired bra will become your mortal enemy – invest in some thin, cotton sports bra-style tops which will give you enough support, but not make you feel like you are going inwardly insane.

EXTRA BEDDING

Especially at the beginning of withdrawal, there are times you are going to need to change your bedding and sheets every single day – sometimes twice if you have a really bad night. Whether it's from the ooze, moisturisers or blood that they will probably be covered in after a long night scratching, you aren't going to want to sleep in them again. If you have some extra bedding ready to go, it will take some of the pressure off trying desperately to get them washed and dried before you need them again.

LOTS (AND LOTS) OF PILLOWCASES

Continuing on from my last point, not only will you need extra pillowcases if you have to change them in the middle of the night, but they can also be very handy in other ways. In the first few months of withdrawal, I found my lower back suffered terribly from oozing, but by putting a pillowcase underneath me, the ooze would mostly collect on there and not on the sheet.

A GOOD VACUUM CLEANER

This will be your best friend through withdrawal and something that you will get to know very well. You will be baffled by how much skin you'll shed through this process and I'm amazed I have any skin left, let alone *good* skin. You will have to vacuum sometimes multiple times a day to keep up with the flakes. Brace yourself and make sure yours is up to the challenge.

KEEP COOL

I started withdrawal through a heatwave and on top of the severe symptoms I was experiencing, it was hell. The desire to keep cool if you are shivery is tough, but sometimes, your skin needs to get as much of the heat out of it as possible, especially if it is angry and red. My mum bought me an electric fan and I can't tell you how much it helped me through withdrawal. When I started, I noticed a lot of people were advising to use ice packs, but as I didn't have a freezer at the time, I would roll a glass bottle filled with water that I had put in the fridge over my skin which was absolute bliss and really took some of the fire out of it. It occasionally worked for the irritation, too, but I don't think there is much you can do when you just *have* to scratch. I also think that a cold water bottle is less damaging than an ice pack – I've used them before, but found them to almost burn your skin and if you have experienced the same issue, I'd definitely try a cold water bottle instead.

DISTRACTION IS KEY

I can safely say that reading and writing got me through withdrawal. Writing kept my hands and mind busy and it was the same with reading. I also found that any time I felt particularly bad, watching something positive or funny really helped. Have a hobby that brings you joy which you can turn to when you need an escape.

SUPPORT

I couldn't have got through withdrawal without my mum, family and friends, but if you are going through this on your own, or your loved ones don't agree with what you are doing, get online and reach out to the TSW community. There, you will find some incredible individuals on both Instagram and Facebook who will support and root for you every step of the way. Don't suffer in silence as there are people out there who care.

SUN

When your skin is strong enough (which for me was after nearly two years of withdrawal), I do believe that getting a bit of sun can do wonders for your skin – but don't do it before you are ready as it could do more harm than good. You will know instinctively when it feels right, so don't overdo it and … wait for it … Give. It. Time.

As you can see, I don't have much to share with you all and your survival kit is looking pretty bare. I have no miracle product or drug which will make this experience any easier, but I would like to give you a word of advice: take away the fear and doubt that you won't get better as without that, you suddenly have something a little more manageable – you have hope, and hope is the most powerful commodity in your arsenal.

6

MY TIMELINE OF WITHDRAWAL

I wanted to create a timeline of sorts which you can use as a guideline to see how I was at certain points of withdrawal. Some of this is guesswork, and I've had to refer to my own photos and information to put all the pieces of my withdrawal together, but I hope you still find it useful.

MONTH ONE
(6th June – 5th July 2013)

Week one

- Within a day or so of starting withdrawal, I had a thin layer of golden crust above my upper lip which I was able to dust off and cover with make-up, and apart from some slight puffiness around my eyes, I was pretty much normal.

Week two

- No more crusty upper lip (I still don't know what that was as it only lasted a few days), but I found I was exhausted all the time and generally not with it.
- Even though my eyelids, lips and face were starting to swell and my skin was dry, I was still able to carry on with my life as normal.
- I was a lot more irritated, but at this point, it was definitely not the bone-deep itch which I experienced through most of my withdrawal.

Week three

- This is where I took a rather sudden turn for the worse. I woke up exactly two weeks into withdrawal feeling extremely uncomfortable and over the next few days, my skin became very red and my eyes were puffy. This continued for the rest of the week and the red skin spread to my neck with patches on my arms and hands.

Week four

- Symptoms continued to worsen.
- I experienced broken sleep and weeping on certain parts of my face like my eyelids and around my mouth.
- I felt totally and utterly wiped out.

MONTH TWO
(6th July – 5th August 2013)

(6th July – 5th August 2013)

- The main areas affected at this point were my face, ears, neck and arms.
- The weeping started on my neck and arms, which were also very itchy and swollen.
- Red patches appeared on my chest, stomach and back.
- I developed full red sleeves with white palms.
- My legs remained unaffected, but the whole top half of my body was red apart from an area on my chest and torso which almost looked like I was wearing a white vest.
- I started feeling shivery and didn't sweat at all, even though the UK was in the middle of a heatwave. Along with the shivering, I also started to feel a little panicky.

- The weeping continued on my eyelids, ears, mouth, face, arms, back and chest – pretty much the entire top half of my body which was so angry and red at times that it looked purple.
- Symptoms spread to my lower back.
- I continued to experience broken sleep and waking up in the middle of the night to scratch – the irritation now felt bone deep.
- At the end of the month, symptoms spread to my legs (not feet) with intense irritation behind my knees and back and the 'white vest' area on my chest and torso filling in with red skin.
- Constant weeping and shedding on a cycle.
- I got a slight infection (I think it was on my legs with some pus-filled spots) so was put on antibiotics.
- After a check-up at the doctors, they said my blood pressure was low.
- This month was when the feeling of burning on my skin really started and didn't let up until I recovered two years later.

~

MONTH THREE

(6ᵗʰ August – 5ᵗʰ September 2013)

- Not as much weeping, but my skin was constantly (and intensely) irritated.
- Bad sleeping patterns.
- I had thick, dry skin with lots of flakes.
- Blood pressure slightly up after a check-up at the doctors and only able to leave the house for my monthly appointment.

~

MONTH FOUR

(6ᵗʰ September – 5ᵗʰ October 2013)

- Blood pressure back to normal.
- Going through a calmer phase, but itching still intense.

~

MONTH FIVE
(6th October – 5th November 2013)

- Showing small signs of improvement and getting more sleep, although itching still intense.
- Able to wear clothes for short periods of time.

MONTH SIX
(6th November – 5th December 2013)

- After a few weeks of improved sleep (although not perfect), back to having problems.
- Found it hard to wear clothes again as it was too uncomfortable and as a result (along with the cold weather), I was unable to leave the house.
- The heating made my skin much drier, but it was hard to turn off when I felt so shivery.

MONTH SEVEN

(6th December 2013 – 5th January 2014)

- Flaring and extremely itchy.
- Clothes still too uncomfortable so I mostly wore cotton pyjama bottoms and nothing else. As I was wearing so little, the heating stayed on most of the time which didn't help with symptoms.
- Towards the end of the month, I showed small signs of improvement.
- It was around this time that I started tapering my moisturiser as I was finding it only irritated my skin more (I have included a full chapter on my Moisturiser Withdrawal experience).

MONTH EIGHT

(6th January – 5th February 2014)

- Continued signs of improvement and getting more sleep, but constantly irritated.
- No weeping at all and not bright red anymore, but symptoms all over my body, including my legs (still not on my feet or

ankles though – gotta take the positives where you can …).

- I flared again.
- Continued to taper moisturisers.

MONTH NINE
(6th February – 5th March 2014)

- Calmer again and showing small signs of improvement.
- Stopped using moisturisers completely.

MONTH TEN
(6th March – 5th April 2014)

- Saw more progress at the beginning of the month, but had another flare with constant irritation and some sleepless nights.
- My skin calmed down again and I managed to get more sleep.

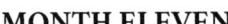

MONTH ELEVEN
(6th April – 5th May 2014)

- Not doing well.
- Skin itchy and sore – I also felt very tired.
- One positive: hair lost through withdrawal started to grow back.

MONTH TWELVE
(6th May – 5th June 2014)

- Flaring.

MONTH THIRTEEN
(6th June – 5th July 2014)

- Making improvements generally, but more localised, severe flaring (very bad on face, hands and neck).
- Getting more sleep at night and even going out for short walks every day.

- Flares more manageable without the weeping and better sleep. Felt more human – unlike the first few months.
- Skin much thicker – before withdrawal it was very thin – and certain areas, better than ever.
- Constant peeling from places I was flaring.
- Later in the month, I got my anniversary flare (which many experience through withdrawal) that exacerbated symptoms on my hands.
- Around this time, with no warning, my left ankle suddenly started flaring badly. I never used topical steroids on that area and to this day, remains a mystery.
- I started excessively sweating, which was extremely painful anywhere the skin was open or dry.

MONTH FOURTEEN
(6th July – 5th August 2014)

- Back and legs completely normal and the skin better than ever.
- Noticeable improvements on my face – swelling down and no puffiness around my eyes.

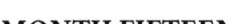

MONTH FIFTEEN

(6ᵗʰ August – 5ᵗʰ September 2014)

- Felt much better in myself and continued to go out on short walks.
- Hands and ankle were the worst places affected and also extremely dry.
- Generally showing real signs of improvement.

MONTH SIXTEEN

(6ᵗʰ September – 5ᵗʰ October 2014)

- Skin up and down with flaring on my hands and ankle.

MONTH SEVENTEEN

(6ᵗʰ October – 5ᵗʰ November 2014)

- Still flaring, but localised and easier to deal with.

MONTH EIGHTEEN
(6th November – 5th December 2014)

- Skin much drier because of the heating and colder weather with constant, localised flaring.

MONTH NINETEEN
(6th December 2014 – 5th January 2015)

- Continued flaring.
- Swollen ankle and hands which would weep intermittently, but a little better when rested.
- Calmer period towards the end of the month.

MONTH TWENTY
(6th January – 5th February 2015)

- Made some progress at the beginning of the month, but things took a turn for the worse and not doing very well at all.

- It was around this time that my mental health really started to go downhill and doubt crept in. A very hard time for me to keep the faith that I was doing the right thing.

MONTH TWENTY-ONE
(*6th February – 5th March 2015*)

- Continued flaring (still localised, but very bad).
- Severe symptoms on my hands, wrists and ankle then generally bad on my face, neck and arms with patches everywhere else.
- To alleviate some of the dryness caused by the central heating and cold weather, I tried using moisturisers again which only made my skin angry, red and even more irritated so I stopped applying them once more.

MONTH TWENTY-TWO
(*6th March – 5th April 2015*)

- Constant localised flaring which continued to affect my mental health very badly.

- Still suffering from swelling on my hands and left ankle which was so swollen at times that I couldn't wear shoes.
- Face and arms still flaring, but not as bad as my hands and ankle.

MONTH TWENTY-THREE
(6th April – 5th May 2015)

- Making some progress and able to go out on short walks again, but my hands and ankle were still very bad.

MONTH TWENTY-FOUR
(6th May – 5th June 2015)

- Noticing small patches of 'normal' looking skin on my hands. Starting to feel positive again.
- Some general improvements and my ankle looking better, too.

MONTH TWENTY-FIVE
(6th June – 5th July 2015)

- Continued to make improvements, but my hands and left ankle were still flaring.
- Symptoms still bad on my face, neck and arm creases.
- Start to think that the sun might be helping with my symptoms.
- Managing better in hot weather and not experiencing the feeling of burning skin as much.

MONTH TWENTY-SIX
(6th July – 5th August 2015)

- More improvements and the excessive sweating calmed down.

MONTH TWENTY-SEVEN
(*6th August – 5th September 2015*)

- One wonderful day in mid-August (Monday 17th August to be exact), I woke up and realised I had recovered from Topical Steroid Addiction.

The AFTER months …

It's daft to continue sharing how my skin has been every single month as, quite simply, there isn't enough to talk about, but since recovering back in August 2015, I have experienced:

- Small, minor rashes on my hands and, very rarely, my face.
- I've noticed if I eat a lot of sugar over a few days or feel like I'm getting a cold, I have dry lips, but it certainly doesn't bother me.
- My hands have flared twice since recovering and both times were when I went to Verbier in Switzerland during months thirty-one and thirty-four. Symptoms only lasted a few

weeks (compared to months in withdrawal) and I'm wondering if it was something to do with the altitude or the fact that I was on a work trip and *certainly* not there for a holiday.

- In month thirty-seven, I experienced an odd bout of hives and was slightly rashy on my chest, torso and back. It wasn't bad at all (and you could barely see anything there), but nevertheless, it brought on a serious case of anxiety. The hives etc. only lasted a few weeks.

- Anxiety marred my life for two years after TSW and any minor rash I got was dissected and analysed until I started seeing symptoms that weren't actually there. At times, the anxiety and fear of flaring was just as debilitating as any of the physical symptoms I experienced during withdrawal.

- I think my hands were a year behind the rest of me in recovering and needed a further twelve months after withdrawal to catch up.

- Around every three months or so, I get odd nerve zaps (like little electric shocks) and the feeling of thousands of bugs crawling over my skin. It only lasts for an hour or so, and there is no evidence of it on my skin, so it doesn't really bother me – only a mild discomfort. Besides, I know it's only my skin repairing itself after years of damage and being suppressed by steroids.

7

AFTER TSW: REBUILDING MY LIFE FROM 'SCRATCH'

*I*t is hard to explain after everything I have told you why Topical Steroid Withdrawal turned out to be one of the best things that ever happened to me, but it was. It was also one of the hardest. I do believe that the most precious things in life come as a direct result of going through times so painful you don't think you'll make it – it's almost as if they are given to you in that order to make you appreciate the good even more. After my sudden recovery, I was nervous – terrified even – of making grand statements like 'I'm healed' (I still am) and so I proceeded with caution in how I went about returning to my old life after two years of self-imposed exile. It's what I wanted at the time – to take a step back from everything – but I didn't realise how much of an impact it would have on me *after* TSW.

I remember I saw my best friend first. Even though

we had these marathon phone sessions all through withdrawal and nothing appeared to be different, I was scared that when we met in person, things might have changed. The moment we saw each other though it was as if that two-year period never existed and our friendship had strengthened if anything. I think one of the things you learn from withdrawal is who your real friends are. I have to say, I was exceptionally lucky. Even though I chose to isolate myself, I was never made to feel like I was missing out – my friends would talk to me on the phone, send me little care packages and tell me I was missed. After meeting up with my best friend, a group of my close friends then drove down to where I lived and we all had a meal together. I remember writing to them all beforehand warning them that plans could change at any moment if I flared again – the fear that this little piece of unbelievable joy wouldn't last and my skin would once more force me to hide away from the world. Thankfully, I didn't need to cancel and had the most wonderful time – I wasn't someone with a skin condition, but simply a woman having a meal with her friends. My friends actually said how well I looked – and I did look well. I looked better than I had done in my life, but at the back of my mind, I was trying not to get overexcited just in case it didn't last. Winter was coming in a few months and I didn't know what that would mean for me and my skin.

At this point, I hadn't left the small town where I

lived – or been on public transport, or even in a car – for well over two years, and I was scared of going anywhere just in case I needed to get back home quickly … and into a bath. One warm Saturday afternoon, a few weeks after recovering, I decided the time had come to take my first step back into the land of the living, and so I got on a bus with my mum to a town about forty-five minutes away and I cannot tell you how wonderful that journey was. We sped through lush fields and country lanes as the sun shone down on me and my memory is one of overwhelming happiness. After that, I made longer and longer journeys until one day, they were trips into London, and I had forgotten that those two years of isolation ever existed.

Around September 2015, I set up my YouTube channel. I had been thinking about doing it for a while, but something always stopped me – I think it was a desire to just switch off and take a step back from everything. Now I had recovered though, I felt the time had finally come to do something as I knew the importance of seeing someone on the other side of withdrawal. I mean, there were plenty of people out there documenting just how tough the process can be – but not many sticking around to show that you do indeed get better. When I was really suffering, there was a woman who uploaded a couple of videos on YouTube for encouragement. She had completely recovered from TSW and I remember watching them all the time – they kept me going ... until one day they were deleted and I nearly had a meltdown. It might seem a little extreme to anyone who hasn't suffered with anxiety, but that simple act of taking down those videos became some kind of John Grisham-style conspiracy in my head in which pharmaceutical companies and those in the medical community were systematically wiping us all out – or perhaps it was just that Topical Steroid Addiction didn't exist after all. It was at times like that where I found it hard to tell myself that I would get better. When something you turned to for support suddenly gets ripped away, it can make you doubt the process. Most people who recover from TSW tend to vanish from the internet and I found that incredibly hard to deal with. *Where did they go? Did they flare again?! Are they OK?!* I desperately wanted to know what happened *after* TSW – do you just get better then everything's OK? PLEASE COULD SOMEONE JUST TELL ME BECAUSE I'M KIND OF HAVING A BREAKDOWN HERE.

I didn't know what to expect after recovering in August 2015. Can you really just 'heal' and be able to move on with your life without a care in the world? It was because of all those questions that I set up my YouTube channel – to assure others that it does get better, but also document the much-neglected *after*, which in my opinion is just as important as the during.

When I started TSW back in 2013, there was very

little in the way of online support for those going through withdrawal. There was a forum, but to be honest, I'd always leave feeling a little depressed. I didn't realise at the time that there were other options available and it was only after recovering that I discovered the Facebook and Instagram communities. I stumbled across the Facebook groups first when I posted my YouTube video there and very quickly, I was part of this amazing network of people. For the first time, I got to know others who had gone through, or were going through, withdrawal. I posted a few more videos, then, as my passion for spreading awareness increased, I set up an Instagram account and blog. My blog soon became my baby – a place to document a part of my life that had completely changed me as a person. On Instagram, I could grow my passion even further and in turn, got to know the most inspiring and kind group of people I had ever 'met'.

For the first few months after recovering, my time was taken up attempting to rebuild my life whilst also working on TSW-inspired videos and blog posts, but it was all done with an air of caution; the ever-present fear at the back of my mind – haunting me – warning me that I could flare again at any given moment. There were times during those first few months where I'd get a rash, no matter how minor, and spiral into such abject despair and anxiety that I would have a panic attack. Every time it happened, I remember thinking this was it – I was going back into withdrawal. There would be this awful sinking in my stomach, a desperate sadness, that this amazing gift I had been given was being taken away from me and as the weather cooled, I really started to panic that I might go back into withdrawal. Because there is such little information out there about what happens next, I was clueless. In November 2015, I was offered a job that completely changed everything and would mean moving back to London. I very nearly turned it down through fear that when I got there, I'd flare and be trapped, but then it struck me one day that I was being absolutely ridiculous and worrying about things that might never happen meant sacrificing the now, and the now is all we have. And so I moved to London, started my new job – which was a shock to the system to say the least – and tried to throw myself into this new life I had created.

In the months after recovering, physically my symptoms were minor and better than I could ever have wished for with only the odd rash, occasional dry lips and two separate flare-ups on my hands which went quickly, but it was the mental symptoms that had a terrible impact on my life *after* TSW. The fear of flaring I experienced during the first few months post-withdrawal decided to outstay its welcome; resting gently on my shoulder and looking down on me as I lived my life, *waiting* for the moment where I would get a rash to strike then taking pleasure in informing me that my brief but blissful respite was over. It took me two years to physically recover from TSW and another two to fully come to terms with what I had been through. This is my problem with using the word 'heal' for TSW. Healing signifies that the wound is gone, but TSW gives you scars; scars you can't see. The worst kind as there is no cream or magic potion to make them better. TSW lays you bare, and it would be near-on impossible to simply walk away unscathed.

Before TSW, I didn't realise that the mind was capable of taking you from feeling the happiest you have ever been to utter desolation within seconds and how seeing what is essentially a rash can suddenly leave you feeling trapped within a black hole you can't escape from. To anyone who thinks Topical Steroid Addiction is just a skin condition, think again – the toughest symptoms happen in your mind, and those are the wounds which can take the longest to recover from.

TSW definitely changed me in ways I wasn't expecting it to. I'm a quieter person now; especially in social situations, much preferring to listen rather than talk. Now, I don't feel the need to fill every gap of companionable silence with words that aren't needed. There are times where I miss the old me – the me who was outgoing and bubbly and on the surface seemed so confident, but that girl also came with baggage – she didn't love herself, had next to no self-belief and stayed in jobs with little to no prospects through a terrible fear of failure and rejection.

Now, well over two years after that magical day where my physical symptoms disappeared, I finally feel at peace – as if that creature resting on my shoulder has decided to fly away to some distant land. That is not to say it won't return, but for now, I *have* now and that is all that matters.

8

YOU SEE A RASH. I SEE...

*T*his chapter is dedicated to the A word: Anxiety. An unseen symptom which can be just as tough, or worse, than the physical. It's hard to imagine, isn't it? You would think there would be no contest between an oozing body part and something as *trifling* as a bit of anxiety. The difference is, you can't ignore anxiety – you can't bathe it, moisturise it or soak it in a concoction of Dead Sea salt and apple cider vinegar to alleviate symptoms. Anxiety is this all-encompassing monster where you become a prisoner of your own mind.

I was not prepared when I went into this process just how much of a devastating impact it would have on my withdrawal. We look at photos of those suffering and are shocked by how bad it can get, but it is also hard, when there are no pictures, to convey just how terrible the mental symptoms are. People ask me, *so you have no scars?* Physically, no. Mentally, I am riddled with them.

My anxiety was bad through withdrawal and would come in these awful waves, manifesting itself in a deep-rooted fear that I would never get better. I was irrational, I suffered from panic attacks and even developed a phobia. I'd see someone flare and my mind would tell me that I was flaring, too, and when I recovered, my anxiety needed a new project to work on – *how can I still affect this woman if she looks better? I know...* Now, my anxiety was armed with all the memories of what came before and decided to hurt me again by sharing what *could* happen. As a result, after TSW, when I'd see a small, harmless rash, it inevitably came with some big questions attached: WHAT ARE YOU? WHAT ARE YOU GOING TO DO TO ME? PLEASE DON'T HURT ME AGAIN. You're probably thinking, but *surely* it's just a rash. It is never just a rash. To explain it to someone who hasn't been through it, think of a person with a mild skin condition – maybe someone who gets the odd rash during the colder months. *They* will be able to see it for what it is: a rash; something most people in the world get at some point in their lives regardless of their skin. If I get a rash, what do I see? I see over two years of pain, sleepless nights, oozing skin, life snatched away from me ... I have sacrificed many precious days of my life to anxiety. It has taken and never given – a pointless wasteland.

On my blog, I wrote that when I am in the throes of anxiety it feels like I am caught in a tornado; trapped in the centre, my thoughts twisted, and I can't understand what is happening as it is all moving too fast, but then suddenly, it's gone again leaving me shaken and confused. It can come out of nowhere, too, leaving me no time to process my thoughts as my mind is spinning at such an alarming rate and I try to think, to gain perspective, but I can't as I am already swept away by it. It took me just over two years to physically recover from TSW, and a further two to repair what anxiety broke. During that time, none of the rashes I got ever amounted to anything, so imagine what would have happened if anxiety had simply not been there.

What I'd like is for anyone who is currently going through TSW to accept that anxiety is a symptom of withdrawal and nothing more – the booby prize. You are not a weak person for succumbing to it; you are simply human. You can be positive all you like and try to ignore it, but that means ignoring the organ which dictates everything we do: the brain. The only advice I can offer you is to just go with it and keep telling yourself it is not real. Like a child who sees monsters in the cupboard, one day your anxiety – like those monsters – might not be there anymore.

Back in June 2017, Briana, a fellow TSA sufferer, asked me to take part in a documentary she was making about TSW. I said yes in a heartbeat, but wasn't expecting it to have such an incredible impact on me mentally. We filmed over one beautiful summer day in Kent. I met Briana – a wonderful, passionate woman who wanted to make a difference, Kelly (who was still going through withdrawal) and her parents (whose house we filmed in) then Nina and Laura, who had also gone through withdrawal and come out the other side like I had. It was one of those days I will remember for a long time, and I can't tell you exactly how it happened, but when I left that day, the black cloud that had been following me everywhere for over four years waiting to storm was no longer there and hasn't returned since. On the whole, I now see rashes for what they are and try to remember that I have no control over what will happen so I might as well just appreciate every single good skin day I am given.

You are probably wondering by now if there is anything that can be done to ease the anxiety, and even though to an extent you are going to have to ride it out, there are certain things you can do to make it feel a little less scary – and who knows, you might even be able to learn from some of my mistakes, too …

IT IS A SYMPTOM

Before anything, I want to stress the importance of treating anxiety like any other symptom of TSW. For many, it will be a significant part of their journey, whereas for others, it won't, as no person is the same.

RIDE IT OUT

Easier said than done, but continuing on from what I've just said, for the most part, you will simply have to ride it out, grit your teeth and remember IT'S JUST ANOTHER SYMPTOM OF TSW.

THERAPY

This summer (2017), I was offered a free consultation with the wonderful people at The Blue Tree Clinic. From just that one session, I felt so much better and wish I'd been able to have it going through withdrawal – especially afterwards – as it's medicine for your mind. I have said this on my blog before, but I believe the biggest gift of therapy is that it reminds us we are not alone and simply human.

MEDITATION

I discovered meditation about a month after I suddenly recovered from TSW as I was desperate to try anything that might keep my skin so lovely. I went into it feeling a little dubious and came out of it amazed by the impact it had on my mental health. The one drawback of meditation is that it is not a cure for anxiety and needs to be done regularly to really reap the rewards. It acts more like a balm – you could even say a topical steroid – by suppressing the feelings, but life gets in the way and sometimes it's hard to find time for something like meditation. For long term sufferers of anxiety, you need to get to the root cause and find something a little more permanent than meditation, but it certainly does help. I don't know how easy it would be to meditate if you are constantly irritated like I was through withdrawal, but give it a go anyway and see how you get on. You don't need to learn from an ancient guru or go on some life-changing course in Asia to start meditating; I simply found a fifteen-minute mindfulness meditation on YouTube and took it from there. To get you started, I will be including a chapter on my tips for meditation just in case you still find the idea of it a little daunting.

DON'T ISOLATE YOURSELF

Anxiety feeds on isolation and by doing something as simple as talking can have an incredible impact on your mental health. Even someone just holding your hand can break the link between your mind and the way you rationalise and process thoughts.

TELL OTHERS HOW YOU ARE FEELING

You might surprise yourself in how much better you feel by being honest with others and not suffering in silence.

BREATHING TECHNIQUES

This was something I learned in my therapy session. I was taught breathing techniques which you can use when you feel anxiety kicking in. There are plenty available online so do some research and potentially save yourself some sleepless nights.

REMEMBER THAT YOU ARE NOT ALONE

Possibly the most important point to make. Like most things in life, you are not alone and for one problem you think only you have experienced, there will be a million others feeling exactly the same.

I could dress up TSW and make it sound easier than it actually was in a bid to encourage you to go through it, but I refuse to not prepare you for something that will not only affect your skin, but your mind, too. As a society, we have got to start taking mental health seriously as those symptoms could potentially have more devastating consequences.

TSW was a necessary evil which turned out to be one of the best things I have ever done and as I get older, the more I believe that everything happens for a reason.

9

MOISTURISER WITHDRAWAL

To be able to talk about Moisturiser Withdrawal, I think I need to first give you a bit of background so you can fully understand the magnitude of my decision to stop using all moisturisers. As there is so much to cover, I have split this up into two separate chapters: my Moisturiser Withdrawal experience, then some tips, which I believe have helped me thrive for well over two years.

From the moment I was diagnosed with eczema when I was six months old, I was given moisturisers – so we are talking about a story which spans well over twenty-five years. It's an epic tale which ends with the protagonist freed from the at times suffocating clutches of her skincare routine. Over the years I've used creams, ointments, lotions, bath preparations, oils and anything else in between that have been marketed to help 'manage' the enigma that is eczema. There was a period of time in my childhood where it wasn't much of a problem, but when I went to secondary school, aged eleven, my eczema returned and with it came all manner of treatments once more. I remember every doctor's appointment I went to throughout my early teens – I would come out of the surgery clutching a prescription, full of hope that *this* was the cream that would help me. Nothing did of course – apart from steroids, and we all know how *that* relationship turned out.

I remember finding it funny that most labels on my moisturisers said things like, *side effects can include red, irritated skin and rashes*, when in effect they are being used to treat a condition that is essentially red, irritated skin and rashes. When I was a teenager, I was referred to the hospital and initially seen by a nurse called Jeanine who to this day, is the BEST person I have ever talked to about my skin ... why? Because she *had* eczema herself. Unfortunately, Jeanine; the nurse of dreams, left the hospital and I was seen instead by doctors and dermatologists who would either tell me to use strong steroid creams and immunosuppressants or throw a new emollient at me to try that they found in that blasted book of theirs which listed all medicines and treatments known to man. This pattern repeated itself throughout my teenage years and amongst other things, I had a course of oral steroids, topical steroids and let us not forget, Protopic. I then went through early adulthood using a mixture of topical steroids and moisturisers every day – all because I thought this was the only way to 'manage' my INCURABLE eczema.

Fast forward to Thursday 6th June 2013 when I made the best decision of my life: to stop using all steroids and immunosuppressants. For the first six to seven months of withdrawal, I used petroleum jelly about four times a day as for me, that felt like the only way I could keep my skin barely functioning. Petroleum jelly was also recommended by many going through withdrawal at the time, but I found the process of using it pretty traumatic to be honest. Amongst other things, it would take ages to sink in, never came out of my pyjamas even after being washed so the material always felt stiff and cold, and it broke my mum's washing machine.

During those early months of withdrawal, I did some rather drastic experiments where I would take the petroleum jelly away and use nothing, but I can safely say the discomfort was unlike anything I've ever experienced in my life, and I would only last a day or so before I'd have to use it again. At that point, I was using petroleum jelly on the entire top half of my body – I was lucky and never had to use it on my legs. I then decided to try tapering, and this is where I had more success. Each week, I would take petroleum jelly away from a small area of my body then the following week, take another area away. I started with the places that were the least affected until I was left only needing it on my face and hands; the two areas I suffered from TSA the worst. When I got to that point, I was in a bit of a stalemate; I found I was too scared to take petroleum jelly away from those areas as I still felt like I needed something so instead, I decided I would use lighter, more natural creams before taking the final plunge to being totally moisturiser free. I weaned myself down to shea butter (which wasn't brilliant but did the job OK) then after that I tried coconut oil, but because my skin hated it, I thought there was no time like the present and from then on, I was able to completely withdraw from using all moisturisers. I think this all happened around February/March 2014 and looking back, I wish I had written down the exact dates.

For a while, I remember my skin was happier when I used nothing on it. I was very dry and still had pretty tough symptoms from TSW, but knew I was better off without anything and was seeing lots of improvements. Things changed when I hit my anniversary flare in June/July 2014 where amongst other things, my hands went to a whole new level of bad and my left ankle suddenly started flaring terribly. To make matters worse, when the colder weather hit the UK, my skin was so dry. For months, I resisted using any moisturiser as I knew I would be worse off, but around February/March 2015, my mum was really worried about the deep cracks in my skin and how they would increase my chances of infection. At this point, I thought I would at least *try* using moisturiser again to see if it could help because I was really suffering. For the first few days things seemed OK, but it didn't take long for my skin to need more and more cream to achieve the same level of moisture. My skin was also getting extremely irritated and inflamed and rashes were spreading to areas that had been pretty much back to normal for months. During that short period of time, I tried quite a few generic high street moisturisers which had the same effect on my skin.

In March 2015, I decided I was better off without moisturisers (again) and as I had only been using them for a short time, and because I was just so irritated, I didn't even bother gradually withdrawing – I just cut them out completely. After that, things slowly improved. The redness and irritation brought on from using moisturisers again pretty much disappeared straight away and since then – bar my legs (because of shaving) and very rarely, my lips – I haven't used a single thing to moisturise my skin. Now, my skin moisturises itself and any issue I've experienced has been directly related to TSW and nothing to do with needing moisturiser – even better, I sometimes get a greasy scalp.

This is all still a work in progress, and I may feel that one day I need to use moisturisers again properly (hello winter!), but at this moment in time, my skin is happiest when I use nothing on it and just leave it alone. On the days where I don't need to shave my legs, my routine consists of getting out of the shower, putting deodorant on and getting dressed – that's it. It's still such a novel experience for me after a lifetime being restricted by what I could and couldn't do. Back when I had eczema, I used to dream of being one of those people who could do something like swim in the sea on holiday then get out and let the sun dry their skin and not have to immediately slather themselves in moisturiser to feel comfortable again. Now, I could actually do this if I wanted to. Going back, I would love to have seen what would've happened to my eczema if I had just left it alone and let any rashes I had dry up on their own, like I do now, but hindsight is a pointless exercise, isn't it?

To anyone who is unsure what to do for the best, you've got to do what feels right for YOU. There is no right or wrong answer and not everyone will benefit from Moisturiser Withdrawal so trust your instincts.

10

TIPS FOR MOISTURISER
WITHDRAWAL

*C*ontinuing on from the last chapter all about Moisturiser Withdrawal, here are some tips and tricks that I think have helped me use next to no moisturisers and actually thrive for well over two years. I would like to say again that Moisturiser Withdrawal won't be for everyone – we are all different and this is only my personal experience. If you feel your skin could benefit from Moisturiser Withdrawal, then I do hope you find these tips useful.

TAKE MOISTURISER AWAY SLOWLY OVER TIME

I talk about how I did this in the last chapter, but in a nutshell, I tried to stop using moisturiser many times through TSW by going cold turkey, but it was awful, and I always gave up after a day or so. By taking them away slowly, I was able to give my body time to adjust to such a drastic change. For a while, it's not going to feel like skipping through a field of daisies, but it was bearable and for me, it was the right decision for MY skin.

COVER YOUR SKIN AGAINST THE ELEMENTS

Just before winter hit the year I recovered in 2015, I was really worried how my skin would cope with the cold weather, so I decided I would try to keep my skin covered as much as possible and would always wear gloves when I went out and wrap a scarf around my face. I'm not sure if doing any of that helped, but for the whole of winter that year, I didn't feel like I needed to use any moisturiser. The following summer, because I think I have an allergy to an ingredient found in most sun creams, I wanted to find something lightweight to cover my face from the sun and came across something called a Choob. They can be found in most outdoor retailers and are absolutely brilliant. Because they are designed to protect your face, they stay where they are meant to (unlike regular scarves). They are also very comfortable and you can still breathe whilst wearing them. I will warn you now that people's reactions when you have one on are absolutely priceless and without fail, at least one person will ask if you are about to rob a bank – but remember, this is about you and no one else. It's YOUR skin. Now, I still try to keep my face protected where possible – whether it's from hot or cold weather – but over time, my skin has become stronger, more resilient, so there is less of a need to and as a result, I'll probably resemble a leather handbag by the age of forty.

AVOID LONG, HOT SHOWERS/BATHS

I know that sometimes nothing feels better than a long, hot shower or bath, but it will dry you out. In the early months of TSW, or when you're really suffering, by all means have a long, hot shower or bath as it's not going to change things and you need as much comfort as you can get … but if you are serious about doing Moisturiser Withdrawal long-term and want to see some results, I'd definitely turn down the heat and cut the time you spend in hot water. Now, I have a short, warm shower pretty much every day and very rarely take baths.

PAT YOUR SKIN DRY AND NEVER RUB

This is a continuation of my last point, but try where possible when you get out of the bath or shower to gently pat your skin dry opposed to rubbing. I think small changes like this can really make a massive difference.

AVOID CLEANING (HOW FABULOUS!)

Last year especially, I found that my skin really didn't like it when I cleaned or came into contact with cleaning products which contained a lot of chemicals. Pretty much straight away, my lips would start to tingle before drying right out and my skin overall felt slightly irritated. Oddly enough, my mum experienced the same problem with her lips, too. Something I have found to be extremely beneficial that I still do (and love) to this day is to wear cotton gloves under my rubber gloves every time I need to use them. It creates a soft, protective barrier which I cannot recommend enough. I get mine at Boots, but they sell them practically everywhere worldwide.

DON'T LICK YOUR LIPS

Try not to lick your lips – especially if they feel dry or irritated as it will only make matters worse. I realised a few years ago that when I concentrate hard on something, I press my lips together or lick them. Even now, I'm still trying to get out of the habit of doing it as my lips can occasionally get chapped or sore if I've eaten too much sugar or have a cold, so it can be like rubbing salt into a wound.

DON'T OVER-WASH YOUR HANDS

I hasten to add that I don't go around with dirty hands, but I am very conscious of how much I wash them. We all know that soap dries out the skin – so does repeatedly putting your hands in water. When I *do* wash them, I'll use a sensitive soap from Dove that I absolutely love as it's so gentle (which I talk about in a chapter all about my current beauty routine post-TSW). I try to avoid where possible using stronger, perfumed soaps as I tend to find they really dry out the skin on my hands, especially if I use them over a prolonged period of time.

TURN OFF THE HEATING

I think you are inevitably going to experience some kind of reaction to colder weather, especially when mixed with any kind of heating – most people do. I always find that my skin, even now, is much drier during the colder months, but notice an even bigger difference when I use an electric fan heater as opposed to central heating. Electric fan heaters spew heat directly into the atmosphere and onto your skin which is much harsher, whereas central heating warms the air through pipes and radiators so the heat is contained. Either alternative isn't great so try where possible to use layers instead of any kind of artificial heat.

KEEP HYDRATED

Apart from when I go out socially, the only two things I'll ever really drink are water and green tea. On an average day, I'll have two to three cups of green tea after meals which I love then drink water the rest of the time. Instinctively, I have always drunk a lot of water and tend to consume around two litres a day. I would like to state that I am six foot and lead a very active lifestyle so that amount of water feels right for me, but might not necessarily be good for you.

I feel like I need to add that I have never liked coffee and in the last few years, I've read a lot of reports about it drying out your skin, so it might be worth cutting out to see if it makes a difference.

A BALANCED DIET

Now this is where I think diet can really make a big difference. I may not believe that food can 'heal' Topical Steroid Addiction, but I do think that a healthy, balanced diet can do wonders for the overall quality of your skin. I try to have an avocado every day and eat oily fish three to four times a week. There are many studies about how refined sugar can affect your skin negatively and I couldn't agree more. Now, I find that when I have too much refined sugar, it tends to dry out the skin on my lips. If you have ever looked at my Instagram account then you will know I definitely haven't cut it out, but I try to avoid it where possible. I have also never taken any supplements as I prefer getting nutrients from the source if that makes sense. I hope I don't offend anyone reading this, but I do not believe that supplements are good for you – that is only my opinion, and I am sure there are countless studies out there which prove me wrong.

LISTEN TO YOUR BODY

It sounds so simple, but if you take the time to listen to what your body needs, it will tell you. I say this a lot, but you've got to do what feels right for YOU.

Of course, like all things to do with our particular under-researched iatrogenic condition, this is all guesswork, but I would be curious to know what would happen if I didn't apply all these tips to my life … and I don't think it would be good.

11

TSW THROUGH THE EYES OF A PARENT (PART ONE)

I can safely say that I couldn't have got through withdrawal without my mum, Elaine. While it might be you who is experiencing extreme pain and discomfort, those closest to you are also suffering, but in a totally different way and can see what is happening from a unique perspective, so I thought it might be interesting to get her view on things as I knew she kept a diary from the first month of withdrawal. When I read it, I was shocked it was ever that bad – and this was before things really went downhill. This is the first of four chapters by my mum, which I hope those going through withdrawal, and their carers, find useful.

~

CARA WARD

THURSDAY 6 JUNE 2013

On 6 June 2013, my 25-year-old daughter decided to stop using topical steroid cream. I think I set the ball rolling and at this stage I don't know how I feel about that. On the morning of 6 June, I could see the veins through her skin on the lower half and side of her face. I had mentioned that she should think about cutting down the amount of steroid cream she was using in the past, but that morning I had to say something about her skin thinning because I was so worried. She said she was OK, but later that day she decided to look up addicted to topical steroids on the internet and said out of the blue that she was never using them again. I was surprised and glad, but thought she would do it gradually even though I knew she had tried this way before and her skin flared up as soon as she stopped. I now know that it is not eczema that is flaring, but the reaction of the skin without steroids. She said she was going 'cold turkey' and said it was the only way because any amount of steroid use just keeps the problem going. She was very determined and I said I would help her in any way I could.

FRIDAY 7 TO WEDNESDAY 19 JUNE 2013

Over the next twelve days her lips became swollen and slightly open underneath and her skin was dry. She had patches appear on her arms where steroid cream had not been applied. Strangely the patches of 'eczema' on her wrist and knuckles didn't get too much worse at that time. Her skin didn't look too bad and she felt OK so did four shifts from 13-16 June at work and stayed with a friend for four nights because we live a long way from her work.

THURSDAY 20 JUNE 2013

It all seemed manageable until the early hours of Thursday 20 June when she woke up feeling extremely uncomfortable. I looked for something to fan her with and found a large Ordnance Survey book and that helped to a degree, but then I remembered a glass bottle of water in the fridge and she rolled it over her skin and that really helped.

FRIDAY 21 JUNE 2013

Early evening on Friday we decided to go for a walk and on the way, met a neighbour we hadn't seen before who introduced himself. He had a dog and we both stroked it and didn't really think about it, but she was very itchy during the night. The next morning, her skin was very red and her eyes were puffy. She suggested it could have been stroking the dog that triggered something, but we will never know. I felt very low because I was frightened at the severity of the reaction and I didn't know if she was doing the right thing. I even suggested that she use a little steroid cream to dampen it all down because she looked so uncomfortable. She said no because the way she was reacting made her realise how dangerous steroid cream is. I bought an electric fan for her with four speed settings and that has proved to be invaluable and the best relief for her so far.

SATURDAY 22 AND SUNDAY 23 JUNE 2013

A black weekend from my point of view because I was so worried about her, but tried not to show it because she was dealing with so much. I decided to read online blogs to find out as much as I could and I am so grateful that people shared their stories because I could see that what she was suffering was a common reaction to coming off steroids but that you could get through it. I told her that I was behind her one hundred per cent and that I would help in any way possible. I told her not to think about work and to concentrate on looking after herself.

MONDAY 24 TO THURSDAY 27 JUNE 2013

She had shifts at work booked for 1 and 2 July and was determined to go. I was in the chemist and noticed some hand-held fans for only £1 each and bought 4 for her. To get to work is a two-hour journey on the bus and tube and I thought they would help keep her comfortable. However, from Monday to Thursday she was definitely worse and her skin was very red on her face and neck with patches over her arms and hands and her eyes were puffier. As the week progressed, I told her she shouldn't think about work, but she was still determined to go.

FRIDAY 28 JUNE 2013

She woke up during the night very itchy and uncomfortable and it took a long time for her to go back to sleep.

SATURDAY 29 JUNE 2013

Friday night we went to bed just after midnight and she woke around 2am extremely uncomfortable and tried not to wake me, but I woke up after thirty or so minutes of her being awake. I am usually a very light sleeper so she must have tried to be really quiet. I told her to wake me from now on so she is not alone at night.

She managed to get to sleep around 4am and felt awful when she woke up, but gradually felt a bit better and asked if we could go to the nearest shopping centre because she was getting 'cabin fever' and also wanted to see if she could manage to get to work. Plus, she needed new cotton pyjamas, so we decided to go, but it is almost an hour on the bus from where we live. She felt OK on the journey there, but after a very short time at the shops, felt exhausted and her skin was flaring. We got the pyjamas and came back home. At this point, she knew work was out of the question and decided to let them know that she was taking July off, but would keep them up to date. Fortunately, it is not a problem with her job because it is not permanent and they can get other people to do the shifts.

MONDAY 1 JULY 2013

The worst day so far. She went to bed on Sunday around 11pm and managed to get to sleep after half an hour or so. She slept through the night until 10am, but said as she came through the door 'don't get a shock'. She had an extremely puffy face and her skin must have been weeping through the night on her eyelids, face and badly around her mouth. She couldn't move (or close) her mouth and her eyes were slits. The skin on her face and neck was extremely red and dry. I suggested calling the doctor and she agreed. Unfortunately, the only appointment they could offer was 3.50pm with a doctor my daughter had seen once before when her skin had flared and the 1% hydrocortisone cream she was using didn't have any effect. At that time the doctor was very offhand and suggested a stronger steroid cream, so my daughter said no to the appointment.

She decided to take an antihistamine tablet and I

bathed her eyelids and around her mouth with a cotton pad soaked in warm water and she was able to eat her breakfast, but it took a long time. I keep two cotton pads soaked in water in a covered dish in the fridge for her eyes and replace with new when she uses them. She put the pads on her eyes and had a warm bath. It is 2pm and she feels a bit better and the swelling has gone down a bit, but she feels wiped out.

I decided to do this diary today because it is so difficult to remember exactly when things happen and hopefully it will help other people. Reading this back, it sounds like doom and gloom, but we have occasionally managed to find humour in the situation and at times it has been difficult because she tries not to laugh and crack her mouth where the skin is tight.

12

TSW THROUGH THE EYES OF A PARENT (PART TWO)

As promised, here is another chapter written by my mum. It's all about how she felt after withdrawal and how she found the whole experience.

~

In my mum's words *Written October 2015*

When my daughter asked me to write a follow-up to my diary I said yes and knew what I would say, but sitting down to actually write this is so difficult. The last two years are very hard to describe. They have been so challenging for both of us in different ways. It is lucky that I work from home so I could look after her properly, but I wouldn't have been able to leave her anyway, especially in the first six months.

When things started getting really bad about three weeks in, the initial excitement of knowing that Cara could be free from steroids turned to fear. Her face was swollen, her skin was weeping including her ears and I was so worried about her. Reading blogs and watching videos helped, but it was still so new, and I was worried that Cara might be an exception. I am so glad she was strong and that the decision to carry on was out of my hands. All I could do was support her and make her as comfortable as possible.

I bought lots of bedding because sheets and pillowcases had to be changed every day (and sometimes during the night) due to weeping skin. Neither of us got a lot of sleep during the first year. Because her hands were so bad, I washed her hair and had to do quite a lot for her physically that she was unable to do. I had a routine every day and worked long hours which stopped me thinking too much about what was happening.

It is difficult to explain to people what TSW is. A friend of mine who has known Cara since she was a baby popped in one afternoon and when he saw her he was very upset and said afterwards that she looked like she had been badly burnt.

Looking back now, it's all a bit of a blur and I am so glad Cara took photos because it would be difficult to remember just how bad it was.

Cara wanted me to write about my experience and all I can say is that I have found out I am stronger than I thought. I felt a bit desperate at times, but got through it, and I appreciate everything now. I have found out so much about Cara and myself and it has changed us both for the better. It was a long road (26/27 months), but it is wonderful to see her so well now. She might flare again, but she is enjoying the simple things like having a quick shower and getting dressed, walking outside in all weathers without being uncomfortable and not thinking about her skin. I do a double take sometimes when I look at her because she looks just like she did before she started TSW and I was beginning to think that would never happen. Also, her skin is better than ever now and a creamy colour whereas before TSW, I realise it had a bit of a grey tinge to it.

I hope TSW and TSA are taken seriously by all doctors soon. About 4 months ago, an age spot I had on my hand became red and angry and changed shape. I left it for a few weeks, but it didn't get better. I went to the doctor and he said he would give me a cream and if it didn't work, to go back. I asked if the cream was a topical steroid. He said it was and I said that my daughter was going through Topical Steroid Withdrawal and she wouldn't be very happy to have it in the house. He winked and smiled and said, 'Don't tell her'. I just walked out of there stunned, didn't get the cream and the spot cleared up on its own.

To anyone going through TSW, and carers looking after TSW sufferers, especially those with young children, my heart goes out to you and I am sending you a big hug xx

13

FROM MY MUM'S PERSPECTIVE: MY DAUGHTER'S ECZEMA HISTORY AND MY VIEW ON TOPICAL STEROIDS

This is the penultimate chapter from my mum's perspective. It is all about my eczema history and her view of steroids which might help parents with young children who have eczema especially. I found it hard to read as it brought up certain unpleasant memories. I really hope that one day the treatment of eczema is changed because it is simply not working and only causing other problems like TSA.

~

In my mum's words *Written October 2015*

I think Cara's eczema started when she was just over 6 months old. I remember she had a small patch of dry skin on her wrist and I mentioned it at the baby clinic. I was told that it looked like eczema and that I should take her to the doctor. I did and hydrocortisone was prescribed for her. I read the label and was reluctant to use it, but I did, and more patches came up all over her body. That was the start of years of doctor and hospital appointments and countless prescriptions for various strengths of topical steroids in cream and ointment form with some containing antibiotic and antifungal agents. I also had a cupboard full of emollients and products to use in the bath.

At the time, I was told eczema was incurable, so joined the National Eczema Society. I bought the NES Christmas cards every year and sold stickers in Brent Cross with my mum helping to raise money for research, hoping that a cure would be found because seeing my daughter so uncomfortable was heart-breaking. After her bath, I would use the prescribed creams and emollients and her skin would come up red and angry. I did what I was supposed to be doing, but it didn't seem right to me. I was told that she mustn't scratch because she could be open to infection and that it thins the skin, so bought cotton all-in-one pyjamas with covered hands and feet that I found out about from the National Eczema Society. They were very expensive – I think about £25 each. She only wore them for a very short time because it was like seeing the person you love itchy in a straightjacket – torture.

I applied topical steroids only when absolutely necessary and very sparingly and Cara's skin was not too bad during the latter part of her time at primary school. She was very happy and loved school.

When Cara started secondary school, her skin became really bad again. She was extremely unhappy at school and started to have regular appointments with a dermatologist at the hospital. I would go with her before school and I have to say that it was a very unpleasant experience. The doctors we saw would get very irritated that her skin wasn't improving and said that we were not using the prescribed creams correctly. One doctor was so bad I told him that Cara was being bullied at school and didn't need to be bullied by him, too. He apologised and said that because she was so stressed it was probably making her skin worse. There was a ray of sunshine at the hospital in the form of a nurse who had eczema. She gave Cara some good tips and really understood what it was like to live with a skin condition.

Cara's skin became so bad in her mid-teens that she was prescribed oral steroids. I think it was a three-month course and she had to carry a card with her for a year after saying that she had taken them. I really didn't want her to take them and felt that she was pushed into it to some degree. Cara also took a lot of antibiotics during her teens because her skin became infected regularly.

Looking back, I think I know what may have caused a reaction in Cara's skin at 6 months old, but of course I can't be certain. I breastfed Cara for 14 months in total, but started to give her cow's milk at 6 months and I think her skin was reacting to that. With hindsight, and everything I know now, I would have stopped giving her cow's milk and left the small patch of 'eczema' alone.

~

My thoughts on Topical Steroid Withdrawal:

It should never get to the point where TSW is required. I think topical steroids are over-prescribed and you can also buy them over the counter. It says on the leaflet to only use them for a short time and under the close supervision of a doctor. If statistics are anything to go by, how can that ever be monitored? People have to study/work/look after children etc. and are caught in a cycle of using steroids in order to function while building up another skin condition along with other problems that will come to a head sooner or later. I don't know what the answer is, and have no medical training whatsoever, but feel that when skin becomes inflamed, it is an indication that something isn't working properly on the inside.

14

A DIARY OF TSW THAT I NEVER THOUGHT I HAD

his is the last chapter from my mum which I am very excited to be able to share with you all. It is an invaluable insight into my withdrawal made up of snippets from email conversations my mum had with her friends over my two-year withdrawal, updating them on my progress. It was my mum's idea, and I am so glad she did it, as I had forgotten certain things that happened and even remember some parts differently. It also made me realise just how tough it was for those two plus years as I had been beginning to wonder if it really was as bad as I thought. Some of the entries have been pieced together from separate emails to other people, there are also replies from the same day, and some are only sentences, but I think it will help you get a pretty good idea of what it was like for me at the time.

I hope it gives you a little injection of hope that you

will get better. TSW is incredibly scary and confusing and can feel at times like it will never end, but it does. Use this diary as a reminder that anything can happen at any given time. It's very long, so either grab yourself the largest mug of tea known to man, or save it for a later date.

~

23 JUNE 13

Cara has been relying on steroid cream to treat her eczema, but after finding out about something called Topical Steroid Addiction, she has decided to stop using it and go 'cold turkey'. Needless to say, she has had a major flare up and it has knocked her out. She has had to miss shifts at work and is taking it one day at a time. It is going to be a rough ride for her, but she is determined to do something about it now.

1 JULY 13

TSW can take 6-24 months before you are healed and the withdrawal effects are severe. Cara stopped on 6 June and it wasn't too bad in the beginning (compared to what we had seen online) – slight weeping below her mouth, extremely dry skin and red patches on her arms and she managed to do some shifts at work and stayed with a friend for four nights. It started to get a lot worse from 20 June and she wakes up in the night very uncomfortable. Her face and neck are bright red, her eyes are puffy and the skin on her face is weeping. Today is definitely the worst day so far. I am very worried about her, but have looked at blogs of people also going through this all over the world and the symptoms are the same, but they eventually heal. I am letting you know this because if she is not too good on 11 July, I won't leave her.

2 JULY 13

Cara is in a bad way. Last night was the worst night so far. I am attaching a link to a video by a doctor who recognises steroid addiction. She is determined to do this and all I can do is support her and make her as comfortable as possible, but I am thinking of making an appointment with a doctor today and tell them what is happening and see if they will just let her come in for a check-up now and again. It is so good just to type it out so thank you for listening. I can be strong if I know no harm will come to her. There are so many blogs of people who are coming off steroids and they are going through hell. It makes you realise that special creams or taking various foods out of your diet (dairy, wheat, sugar etc.) will make no difference while you have steroids in your system.

I have made an appointment with the doctor for Thursday morning, but will phone at 8am tomorrow to try to get an earlier appointment. We have no idea what is going to happen next with her skin and how long it will take to heal. I was reading about a young girl yesterday and it has taken her over two years to get over it, but it could be 6 months, we just don't know. I have been wary of topical steroids because they can cause thinning of the skin, but wasn't aware that when you stop using them you have withdrawal flares as your skin has become addicted to them.

3 JULY 13

Cara had a bad night with not much sleep, but the puffiness is down a bit so that is making her feel better. Hopefully she is starting to go through a better phase so she is more comfortable.

5 JULY 13

We saw a doctor yesterday who was very kind and wasn't horrified by what she is doing. He prescribed a very strong antihistamine with a sedative so she could sleep at night. Cara has never had a problem sleeping until now because she is so irritated. She looked it up as soon as she got home and really doesn't want to take it because it can cause other problems. She wants to try to get through it without adding other medication if possible. We both wanted a doctor on board in case of complications because this is a relatively new thing and we only have info from what we have seen on the internet. To be honest, if it wasn't for the wonderful people blogging and taking photos of what happens, I would have been a nervous wreck because it really is brutal to witness, but I know from them this is normal for withdrawal and Cara is coping with it. All I can do is support her in any way and her friends have been wonderful.

7 JULY 13

Cara is going to try to eat a very plain nutritious diet. For now, I have been concentrating on vitamins A, C and E for Cara, but we need to rethink everything. We are looking into giving up milk – at the moment we both love porridge and blueberries for breakfast so looking at alternatives for the milk. Cara's skin weeps on her neck and face and last week her skin was so dry that the skin cracked along a fold of her neck. It was quite bad, but healed very quickly which surprised me even though she has always had fast healing skin so very grateful for that.

9 JULY 13

The hot weather isn't good for Cara, but she has an electric fan now which helps. We have cut out sugar (apart from natural sugars) and it hasn't been hard, but that might be due to the hot weather. Cara has been having Greek yoghurt every day and hasn't had wheat since Saturday and has noticed a difference in a good way after that short time.

10 JULY 13

Cara had a bad day yesterday, but today seems a bit better and the cooler weather helps. It will be a relief if this is the answer to finally forget about eczema and allow her to have a better quality of life.

11 JULY 13

It's five weeks today since Cara stopped using steroids. She has taken a photo of herself every day since Saturday 29 June to record the changes. The main parts affected are her face, ears, neck and arms and they are very red and weep and are extremely itchy. She has patches on her chest, stomach and back. Her arms were swollen, but they have gone down now thank goodness and the puffiness has gone down in her face apart from her eyes. I bought an electric fan because it has been very hot here for the last week and that really helped. We don't really know what will happen because looking back at the photos, they are different every day.

Cara is eating an avocado every day, oily fish, plain probiotic yoghurt with fruit, green vegetables and carrots, extra virgin olive oil on potatoes and salads and porridge with blueberries for breakfast.

15 JULY 13

Cara isn't sleeping well at all. It is very common with other people going through the same thing and they seem to average 2-3 hours a night. Yesterday was awful. I felt so emotional all day and just wanted to cry. Cara takes a photo every morning to record the changes and looking at them last night was just so sad. It is the strangest thing because it is so changeable. My sister in America is being very supportive and sent her a lovely email and Cara speaks to her friends on the phone. I'll have to go because I have lots of work to catch up on, but will email during the week to let you know how she is.

17 JULY 13

Our flat is very hot and difficult to cool down even with an electric fan. Cara is finding it very difficult and sleeps only a couple of hours a night. She is not too good at the moment and we don't know if the heat is making it worse. She has an appointment with a doctor 'with a special interest in dermatology' on Friday, but we both think she is not up to the journey so might have to cancel. Cara thinks it is pointless going anyway and she has an appointment with the local doctor next week who can check she is OK. There is no real treatment for this and it should get better with time.

Cara was very uncomfortable last night before bed, but managed to calm down and slept a bit longer than the night before.

18 JULY 13

I bought an electric fan a few weeks ago for Cara and it really helped her in the beginning with the itching, but she tries not to put it on too much because it dries out her skin even more. It has been so hot here and it has been really bad for Cara. The bedroom is an attic room with a small window that is protected either side so no air gets through and during the night it was stifling even with the electric fan. A couple of nights ago, I brought the mattress downstairs to the living room and it is cooler because there are two windows at each end of the room. A positive of the hot weather is that I am doing a lot of washing every day and it dries really quickly. Cara has all the symptoms of TSW now. Her skin is very red and she has red sleeves and white palms. Her legs are not affected, but her upper body is red apart from a white 'vest'. Last night, she became a bit distressed and felt shivery even in the heat. If I didn't know that this was normal for TSW, I would be frantic, but have to help her as she is determined and I don't think there is any other way. Looking forward to cooler weather because that will definitely help her.

Cara cancelled her appointment with the doctor at the hospital because the journey would be too much for her and she doesn't think it will do any good. She has an appointment with the local doctor next week.

Cara only wears cotton pyjamas all day – very loose T-shirt style with short sleeves, but mostly has the top off. I use non-biological powder and don't use very much. Cara doesn't really sweat much which is to be expected, but her skin should perform normally one day. She has been taking over-the-counter antihistamines, but doesn't overuse them so they are effective when she needs them.

19 JULY 13

I am attaching a photo Cara took this morning of her arm. Looks paler in the photo than it actually is in real life, but you can still see the contrast.

22 JULY 13

Cara has had a bad couple of nights. It is very changeable, but is to be expected from what we have seen other people go through.

25 JULY 13

Just got back from the local doctors with Cara. She is going every month (or before if she needs to) so he can keep an eye on her. He took her blood pressure and said it was low and that was good. He said he was very interested in what she is doing and is using her as a case study. I am just glad he knows the situation and Cara said she will tell me if she needs help. I will help and support her in any way I can, but it is a bit scary at times. Cara told him she didn't get the prescription for the strong antihistamines with the sedative he gave her last month because she wants to get through it as naturally as possible.

27 JULY 13

Cara has gone down a notch this week – she gets shivery and a bit panicky for a while, but manages to calm down. Her skin is so angry and red (looks purple sometimes) and it has spread to her lower back badly and she is very uncomfortable. Her face and arms weep and she wakes in the night to scratch. I don't want to leave her at all to go anywhere other than the local shops so I ordered another sheet and some more cotton pyjamas online from M&S and they arrived yesterday so that will help with having enough to change now.

I think any form of relaxation will help and Cara is going to try breathing slowly if she feels a bit overwhelmed. My friend has just visited and Cara said she didn't mind seeing him. When I saw him out, he said he was shocked and a bit upset because he has known her for years and said it looked like she had been burnt.

Cara is a member of a TSW forum and she is doing a lot of research when she is not feeling too bad. She doesn't feel like reading at the moment. Hopefully she will have a calmer period soon to recharge her batteries. It has been raining for about half an hour so that should freshen everything up.

It's strange you should say that about the forum because Cara has said that the majority of the posts are not very positive and a bit bleak, but she mainly looks at it for information. She enjoys watching Ellen and when she is not feeling too good, she looks at Persian kittens on YouTube. I suggested very simple yoga might be good for her when she is feeling better. A few weeks ago, I got her an audio book from the library because I thought it might distract her at night, but her skin gets so irritated that any noise adds to it and she can't concentrate.

Cara has just gone to have another bath. I sometimes get a little frightened because so few (it seems) people have gone through or are going through withdrawal from steroids and it looks so bad that I just hope she will be OK. I can be very strong if I know she will be OK in the end and just have to trust that she will be. It is so good to be able to write down how I feel and hope you don't mind.

I saw your other email re cotton gloves. I bought some for her when she wasn't too bad at the beginning and taped them loosely around her wrist so she couldn't pull them off in the night (Cara's suggestion) and they worked, but the itch is so intense now that she has to scratch. I am worried about her damaging her skin, but they all scratch and the people who have healed seem to be OK. She cuts her nails very low and doesn't have scratch marks like some people, but her skin weeps. I have been wondering if the scratching helps the healing. The reason we have a tickly cough is because the body is trying to get rid of bad stuff and I wonder if the itching, scratching and weeping is a healing process. I have to try to think of it in a positive way because nothing will stop her scratching.

28 JULY 13

Yes, I agree with you re scratching and infections and it is my biggest worry in all of this. We talked about this with the doctor and Cara knows the signs and can contact him if she needs anything. I just mentioned to Cara your suggestion re gauze and I think she will try it – I will get some tomorrow. We read about this and I think she was a bit worried about the gauze drying on the skin then having to pull it off.

Her skin is so bad at the moment – her arms are swollen and her eyes were very puffy again today. She is weeping from her eyes, ears, mouth, face generally, arms, back and chest – in fact all over. She doesn't complain and it is a bit scary for me at times, but I don't show it because she is coping with so much.

29 JULY 13

Cara was using a loyalty card to scratch and I was keeping it clean. She then tried a large plastic comb with wide set rounded teeth and has been using that and finds it effective. Night time is worse for her. I usually manage about 4-5 hours' sleep in total, but couldn't sleep last night and she was awake most of the time. She tries not to disturb me, but I have told her to wake me because she must feel desperate. She is sleeping now but will probably be up soon and I am catching up with work.

31 JULY 13

Attaching a couple of photos from Monday. The photos don't show how red it is. It has spread to her legs and we are hoping it won't spread to her feet. She is still weeping and shedding lots of skin and not sleeping, but she is trying to stay positive.

1 AUGUST 13

She does have a line on her chest where the redness stops, but her torso is gradually filling in. It started with her lower back and is creeping up. She doesn't have blisters – it looks like that, but it is flakes of dry skin and her skin weeps then dries up then weeps again.

Last night after work we watched Jonathan Creek then I massaged Cara's back and arms where she is holding some water. I do it very gently and massage towards the heart. She was very relaxed and managed to sleep more last night so I will do it just before she goes to bed from now on. She feels a bit better today and we don't know if it is the natural course of things and a flare is dying down a bit or if anything we are doing is helping. It is 8 weeks today since she stopped using steroids. There are millions of prescriptions given out each year for topical steroids and 1% hydrocortisone and Eumovate are available over the counter, but relatively few people around the world are going through withdrawal it seems and I just wonder what will happen in a few years' time as more people find out about it.

Have just been to Sainsbury's and it is definitely the hottest day so far. Cara hasn't moved much in the last couple of months, but because she feels a bit better today, she walked up and down the stairs a few times to help her circulation.

3 AUGUST 13

Cara is on antibiotics at the moment because her skin became a bit infected yesterday.

18 AUGUST 13

Cara is in a strange place with this at the moment. Her skin hasn't been weeping for the last couple of weeks, but it has become increasingly itchier and is almost constant. I don't know how she manages to deal with it. The comb is working for her because it isn't breaking her skin, but her skin is extremely dry. I ordered some organic shea butter for her, but it is not moisturising enough and the only thing she can use on her skin to keep it from cracking is petroleum jelly. Cara stopped using steroids ten weeks ago last Thursday and she is staying positive. It has been good to see the blogs of people going through withdrawal who were not in a good place when Cara started and are now starting to see improvements or are more or less healed.

21 AUGUST 13

We have got Epsom salts in because some people mentioned it in their blogs and I thought it might be good for Cara further down the line. Sleep is still a problem and we are keeping very odd hours at the moment. We usually get to bed around 1.30-2am and wake on and off during the night, but we are going to try to get to bed earlier tonight because Cara has got her monthly appointment with the doctor at 9.10am tomorrow and she needs to put petroleum jelly on 1-2 hours before we leave. Can't believe it is a month since we were last at the doctors.

22 AUGUST 13

Cara saw the doctor this morning and her blood pressure was up slightly, but still normal so that is good. He was again very sympathetic and interested in what she is doing. She is shedding lots of skin at the moment and he offered her something for the bath, but she insists on not having anything chemical and I think he agrees with her. He said she can contact him if she needs anything and it is so good that he is making a note of everything so she doesn't need to explain the whole thing to anyone else. He also mentioned he had been doing some research and hopefully he will not keep prescribing stronger topical steroids for other patients when their skin condition doesn't improve. She is going to see him again in a month. She was feeling a bit low yesterday (doesn't happen very often) and was worried that she wasn't going to heal, but this morning she feels better again after reading a blog post about a girl who is going through TSW. She is around the same age as Cara and there was a before picture of the girl's hand that looked like Cara's does now then her hand after about 450 days and it looks amazing.

23 AUGUST 13

Been a bit of a tough week for her this week. Her skin is very red and thick and she is shedding skin constantly and extremely itchy but from reading blogs, this appears to be normal for withdrawal. She also had her monthly appointment with the local doctor yesterday – the only time she goes out at the moment.

I certainly couldn't leave Cara at the moment. People can become suicidal doing this although Cara loves life, but this is brutal, and I don't know how she is coping with it. I will be able to leave her further down the line, but it is so hard to say when that will be.

27 AUGUST 13

Cara is almost at the three-month mark and from what we have read, months three and four are quite bad for other people. I don't know how she is managing to deal with the constant irritation all over.

2 SEPTEMBER 13

Cara is not doing too well at the moment. There is not much weeping, but the itching is constant and she isn't getting much sleep. Her skin is incredibly dry and there are flakes of skin everywhere. She is still feeling positive though and her friends are great, keeping in contact a lot.

15 SEPTEMBER 13

We have had a challenging couple of weeks, but Cara has had a few days where she has felt better so is making the most of it.

19 SEPTEMBER 13

Just back from Cara's monthly appointment with the doctor and her blood pressure was normal which is good. She had a really bad time a couple of weeks ago and was very worn down, but is now going through a calmer period – still very itchy though. Two weeks ago tomorrow, it looked like her skin was infected and she was covered in spots. We got a prescription for antibiotics after 6.00pm from the doctor, but the pharmacy was closed. On the Saturday, I took the prescription into our local chemist, but they didn't have them so had to go to further afield. When I got back (it took 3 hours) her skin looked calmer, so she decided to wait until the following day to take them. Her skin was better the next day, so she didn't need to take them and I'm glad now that there was a delay. I think her immune system is fighting back which is a good sign, plus I think the food she eats is helping. It is handy to have the antibiotics in just in case she needs them in the future (hopefully she won't). I have had a bit of a bad back and have decided to wash Cara's pyjamas twice in the washing machine because I think washing and rinsing them in the bath first before putting them in the machine was putting a strain on my back. I will see if it works OK.

Cara is using a large round-toothed comb now which she prefers as it hasn't broken her skin and I think you are right that using the card or the comb has been massaging her and helping to keep the swelling down. It is so difficult to assess how long this process will take because it is so up and down. The weather here changed drastically from very hot to very cold and we have even put the heating on this week. A bit milder today though.

29 SEPTEMBER 13

She has had a bit of relief for the last few days and all she wanted to do was read her book today.

13 OCTOBER 13

It would be lovely to see you, but Cara won't be able to come out for the moment because it is very uncomfortable for her to wear clothes. She is showing small signs of improvement and is getting a bit more sleep which is great. She is seeing the doctor on Thursday (the last month has flown by).

17 OCTOBER 13

Cara saw the doctor today and her blood pressure was better – it was a bit low before.

21 OCTOBER 13

Had a short walk with Cara on Saturday and she went out on her own this morning because her skin is slightly better and she is OK wearing clothes for a short period so that is good.

26 OCTOBER 13

Cara's skin is looking slightly better and she is sleeping a bit more although the itchiness is severe at times.

31 OCTOBER 13

Cara is feeling better in herself due to the fact (I think) that she is getting a bit more sleep, but her skin is so irritated I don't know how she is coping with it.

26 NOVEMBER 13

Cara is showing definite signs of improvement although she is having problems sleeping again. She didn't go to the doctors for her monthly check-up just over a week ago because it is very cold and too uncomfortable for her to wear clothes, so she cancelled it. She doesn't go out at all and I only go to Sainsbury's for food, but I had to go to a shopping centre the weekend before last to buy more pyjamas, bedding and towels as we had to throw away the ones we had that were ruined by petroleum jelly. Cara talks to her friends a lot and they have sent her care packages with books and DVDs – they are so sweet. Her friend who she has known from primary school sent her two romantic historical novels by Judith McNaught that she didn't really think she would enjoy, but she loved them. On 6 December, it will be six calendar months since she started and it is a milestone we are both looking forward to.

27 NOVEMBER 13

Cara managed to sleep a bit more last night, but it suddenly got cold and the heating is making her skin even drier, so we are trying to keep it off as much as possible.

9 DECEMBER 13

It is so difficult to know how long this will take. She could be at a point where she will be comfortable enough to wear clothes and go out within a year with the occasional 'flare' or it could be up to two years.

12 DECEMBER 13

Cara is at the doctors for her monthly check-up this morning and should be back soon. She seems to be having a flare at the moment – skin a bit red and extremely itchy (Cara describes it as a bone-deep itch) and disturbed sleep. We were hoping that it would be a little better in the colder weather, but all Cara wears at home is cotton pyjama bottoms and nothing else because clothes are too uncomfortable, so we have to have the heating on more than we would normally. We looked back at the pictures of Cara when she started and they were so shocking, but it made us realise that she is making progress. A lot of people take sleeping pills, pain killers and other drugs, but they all have quite a bad time anyway and Cara refuses to take anything. She seems to be better at an earlier stage than most and we don't know if it is down to her not taking medication, good diet, her constitution or luck. Sometimes it is difficult to believe she is going to get better, but the alternative is not good, so she is staying positive.

3 JANUARY 14

Cara is showing signs of improvement which is great. We didn't do anything for Christmas and New Year, but we had a lovely time (the first New Year's Eve we have spent together in years).

9 JANUARY 14

Cara is improving and getting some sleep now, but the itching continues. She seems to have made progress compared to other people in some ways, but I now think this will take longer than I first thought. There is no weeping and she is not bright red which is great, but it is all over her body including her legs now and although much better than in the beginning, she is still itchy almost all the time.

12 JANUARY 14

Cara is going through a flare at the moment and is very uncomfortable, but we are hoping she will have some normality by the summer and can see her friends again.

10 FEBRUARY 14

Cara is OK, but very tired.

18 MARCH 14

Cara is making progress, but the itching is very bad sometimes.

23 MARCH 14

Cara is improving, but has had a bit of a flare and some sleepless nights.

24 MARCH 14

Cara had a bit of a flare from about mid-week last week. She is starting to feel a bit better now and managed to get some sleep last night. We saw a video of an Australian man who is 18 months into TSW and he is more or less healed. We have been following his progress (and others) and it is very inspiring and he looks like a different person.

7 APRIL 14

Cara is not great at the moment – her skin is very itchy and sore and she is very tired. She lost some hair (usual for TSW), but it is growing back so that is good.

16 APRIL 14

Cara is not too good at the moment. She spends most of her time reading as it is the only thing that seems to take her mind off it.

10 JUNE 14

Cara is improving. She is getting more sleep at night which I think is really helping and she has been going for a short walk every day. She is finding the heat a bit overpowering though and our flat is very hot in summer.

11 JUNE 14

Cara is up and down, but very positive. She has been sleeping through the night which is huge for her, but her face and hands are very bad at the moment (where she mostly used topical steroids). She lost a lot of hair at the beginning, but it is growing back now and is about an inch long.

15 JUNE 14

Cara is improving, but in the middle of a nasty flare. She is able to deal with it because she is getting more sleep and it is localised (hands, face and neck).

19 JUNE 14

We don't have a clue how long this process will last. Cara has always been quite realistic about how long it would take – about 2 years, and I think she might be right. I never thought it would take this long. She is generally better, but is in the middle of a bad flare. She is sleeping through the night and her skin is not weeping (which for her was the hardest part to take). Also, she is able to manage the flares better and still feels human (unlike the first few months which were very hard). Her skin is now thicker than it was (before she came off topical steroids, I was very worried about how thin it was) and in places, better than ever which is encouraging.

9 JULY 14

Cara's skin is still flaring, though not as bad and is now incredibly dry mainly on her hands, face and neck. The skin is peeling off constantly, but she is starting to look like Cara again. She is not using any kind of moisturiser now because it doesn't help and only makes it worse – lots of people are withdrawing from moisturiser, too.

6 AUGUST 14

Her back is completely healed and using this as a guide she thinks that because her back was the first place to get intensely itchy, it is the first to heal and she will continue to heal accordingly.

In January, she decided to stop using moisturiser and did it gradually – by March she was not using anything. The worst places now are her hands and ankles, but there is noticeable improvement in her face and no puffiness around her eyes. I am starting to believe we don't need moisturiser at all. All these things we put on our body sends messages that we don't need to provide our own moisture. When Cara was little, the doctor prescribed various emollients for her skin (one of them even had sodium laurel sulphate in it!) and when I applied them, her skin always became red and angry and didn't help with the eczema. Plus, it was so uncomfortable for her to be covered in cream under her clothes. I have always had doubts about using emollients for eczema. I think when the body itches you have something that needs to be released just as coughing is the body's way of trying to get rid of something bad.

20 AUGUST 14

Cara is showing signs of improvement :) Her back is completely healed and there is no puffiness in her face. The hair she lost, especially around her hairline, is now about two inches long and will soon blend in with the rest of her hair. She is feeling better, too, and goes out for a walk most days. The skin on her face, hands and ankles is incredibly dry and flaking constantly, but that should improve soon, too.

25 AUGUST 14

It has been 14 months (on 6 August) since Cara started. I thought she would be really bad for about 6 months then gradually get better with the odd flare, but she is just coming out of a bad flare that lasted a long time. The good news is she is starting to show real signs of improvement.

23 SEPTEMBER 14

Cara's skin is slightly raised today so it is up and down, but generally better.

11 OCTOBER 14

Cara is going through a bit of a flare, but still so much better than before.

25 NOVEMBER 14

Cara's skin is very dry because of the heating – the best time for her skin is spring or early autumn.

4 DECEMBER 14

She is not doing too well, but she is keeping her spirits up. I don't know how she deals with it – it must be so uncomfortable. The cold weather and heating are not helping. I have been inundated with work again this week and am struggling to keep up, but also enjoying the challenge and it stops me thinking too much. We are OK though and Cara makes me laugh every day.

18 DECEMBER 14

Was up with Cara Tuesday night because her hands and one of her ankles were swollen and painful, but after resting them completely yesterday, they are slightly better.

5 JANUARY 15

Cara is slightly better this week :)

6 JANUARY 15

I do a short (twenty minutes) yoga for beginners I found on YouTube every other night and it is so relaxing I almost fall asleep in the middle of it. It is for relaxation and strengthening your back and I did it initially because I wash Cara's hair over the bath and my back really hurt, but my back is much stronger and I have no problems now.

11 JANUARY 15

Cara is making some progress. She is hoping to feel well enough to see 'Cats' at the end of the month with her friend.

29 JANUARY 15

She has not been too good for the last couple of weeks. She was supposed to see 'Cats' with her friend on Tuesday this week. My friend offered to drive her to meet him at the Palladium then we would go for a meal for my birthday and pick her up outside after, but she was not well enough even for that. She has been very positive, but it is getting through to her now.

16 FEBRUARY 15

Cara is not doing too well. She seems to be in another bad flare and it is taking a lot longer than I thought. I really don't know how she copes with the constant irritation. Her hands, wrists and one ankle are very bad and then generally bad on her face, neck and arms with patches everywhere else. I think she will start to feel better from the spring when she can get small amounts of sun for vitamin D – that should really help. The people going through TSW who live in Australia seem to do better and I think it must be because the climate is generally better.

8 MARCH 15

Cara is not doing so well. There are times when I am very worried about her and there is nothing we can do about it but wait it out. Also, TSW is a relatively new thing and we don't know the long-term effects of it. Her friends have been great and phone her a lot.

10 MARCH 15

Cara seemed slightly better yesterday, but she woke up today with a swollen hand – hoping it doesn't get infected.

12 MARCH 15

The swelling has gone down and no infection, thank goodness. She was slightly better yesterday so hoping it continues to improve.

24 MARCH 15

Cara's skin is very dry and flaking and her hands and one ankle are very bad – she was going out for short walks and even getting some food shopping when I was busy, but she can't wear her trainers at the moment. I am going to get her some flip flops at the weekend. Small amounts of sun should help heal her skin.

30 MARCH 15

Cara's skin is slightly better on her body, but her hands and ankle are still quite bad.

25 APRIL 15

Cara is making some progress and is going out for very short walks to get some sun when she can, but her hands and ankle are still quite bad.

6 MAY 15

Cara has small patches of skin on her hands that look relatively 'normal' and it is 23 months today since she started so looking more positive :)

18 MAY 15

Good weekend – Cara's skin seems to be improving very slightly each day and her ankle is looking better :)

2 JUNE 15

Cara's skin is improving and we hope any flares will get weaker over time.

7 JUNE 15

Cara is better apart from her hands, left ankle, neck, face and creases of arms. I think the sun is helping.

2 JULY 15

It was a very hot night, but as Cara's skin is so much better, she was OK with it.

6 OCTOBER 15

Her skin is just getting better all the time and has never looked this good.

15

A DAY IN THE LIFE OF A TSW SUFFERER

J thought I would 'shed' some light on what a typical day was like for me at various stages of withdrawal. I'm starting at month two as even though I did experience bad symptoms like puffiness (especially on my eyelids), redness on my face and general exhaustion, with the help of make-up, I was able to live a relatively normal life and innocently thought my withdrawal wouldn't be so bad … until about three weeks in when things suddenly took a turn for the worse and marked the start of a rather crazy couple of years …

≈

• YEAR ONE •

AVERAGE DAY (MONTHS 2-6)

Wake up after a fractured night's sleep, barely getting more than an hour or two in one go. My bed would feel like I was in a sandpit from all the dry skin – I hated it. I would have breakfast before a long soak in the bath. Afterwards, I would use petroleum jelly all over the top half of my body (I found my legs didn't need anything) then wait in front of an electric fan for it to sink in, which sometimes took well over an hour. In the early stages, I felt like I was in a Catch 22 situation – I couldn't function without petroleum jelly so endured the tedious waiting time for it to sink in. By doing that, I was given a brief period where things were bearable before I needed moisturiser again … and so began the whole drying process once more. Whilst waiting for it to sink in, I'd find funny or positive things to watch – total escapism basically and anything that would distract me from what I was going through. After some lunch, there would be another layer of petroleum jelly before letting that sink in then collapsing on the bed for a nap which would usually take me into the early evening. I would then either have some dinner followed by another bath/petroleum jelly party or swap it around depending on how my skin felt. Afterwards, I would normally have a window of maybe a couple of hours where I felt awake/conscious enough to write for a while and incredibly, over months two and three, I wrote my first ever 50,000 word draft of a novel. I lived for the hours I was able to write; they kept me going. I would then usually read for a while before putting the last layer of petroleum jelly on and as I let that sink in, Mum and I would watch something together.

By this point, I was terrified of what was to come: bed. As my bedroom was too hot, the mattress was brought downstairs to the living room which was a little more comfortable. My mum didn't want to leave me in case I needed her in the night so she would stay with me. I would sometimes build up such a fear of sleep and the night that I would sit on the edge of the bed, scared of what would inevitably happen – the hours of endless awake as I scratched myself into oblivion, the sinking feeling as the ooze started, the desperate desire for sleep that wouldn't come. The tossing and turning. I would sleep on extra pillowcases (as towels were too lumpy) to soak up the ooze and had a round-toothed comb down by the side of the mattress to use for scratching, but honestly, nothing hit the spot for me like nails did. Sometimes I would read, sometimes Mum would keep me company, but I tried not to wake her unless absolutely necessary as on top of working from home full-time, she also had this twenty-six-year-old baby to look after. I am astounded what she did for me during withdrawal and I will never be able to adequately thank her for getting me through that period of my life. I would fall into a light sleep every few hours before waking in my sandpit of a bed and have to pull the extra pillowcases off my skin where they had stuck to the ooze. I would then brush the bed down, flip the pillowcases over and try once more to find some sleep that I knew was lost to me.

It's strange, but even though the symptoms during the first few months were horrific, it was the petroleum jelly/moisturiser routine which really took me over the edge. I felt trapped by it, but thought I needed it as that is what I was told would help me ...

My outfit of the day during this time was a pair of 100% cotton pyjama bottoms. I would occasionally wear the top which went with the trousers, but it would inevitably get pulled off – I just couldn't bear the feeling of anything on my skin – so I spent most of my time topless. It is hard to explain how it felt to someone who hasn't experienced it, but imagine a panicky feeling and a perpetual irritation that cannot be suppressed until the item is off your skin completely.

Throughout the day, I would have bursts of intense irritation and would only stop scratching once I'd gotten to the source of the itch. In the beginning, I got into a terrible habit of using a loyalty card to scratch my skin which was an absolute joy, but so bad for me. I remember I had to call the company to say I had lost my card. I also tried using a round-toothed comb which I briefly touched on earlier that was sometimes effective, but I'd almost always revert to my nails (or my mum's). Looking back over my whole withdrawal, I now have quite 'controversial' thoughts on the benefits of scratching which I will be talking about in more detail in a later chapter.

I never went anywhere without tissues to mop up the ooze and will always remember how it felt the moment before my skin started to weep – for me at least, there was almost this sinking in my entire body. During the first three or so months, the oozing on the top half of my body was intense, but after that, thankfully, the only places I experienced oozing were on my hands and left ankle.

I think I could count on one hand the times where I left the house during those first few months and mentally, I didn't really have a coping mechanism as I was so completely and utterly out of it – I was a walking zombie – which in a way was a blessing. I was just too tired to process everything that was happening to me. Those first few months are a bit of a blur now and it is only through having to dig deep to write this book that I've remembered some of the horrors of TSW.

AVERAGE DAY (MONTHS 7-12)

Even though months 7-12 were bad, there was practically no oozing and it was also when I started Moisturiser Withdrawal so two of the things which made the first six months horrific, were no longer part of my life. I noticed areas that were very bad or intensely itchy, like my back and behind my knees, during the earlier months were getting better, but I was still not able to go out much at all as the intense burning and feeling of clothes on my skin was unbearable. I went to a monthly check-up at the doctors, but apart from that, I couldn't leave the house. I used this period of time to expand my knowledge and to read and write. As I left school early, I found there were gaps in my knowledge which I then proceeded to fill. I was constantly exhausted from the lack of sleep, so my progress was slow, but I kept going and ended up changing the way I write and even speak, using words I'd never had in my vocabulary before. I spoke to friends more often and noticed small improvements as time passed. I also went down to one bath a day, but the itching was still relentless, as was the burning.

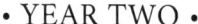

• YEAR TWO •

I am putting this year in one section as I'd call it the stagnant phase where nothing really changed. Sleep returned to me, which made things so much easier, only waking up once or twice in the night, but some symptoms got worse. In month twelve/thirteen, I got what I think was my anniversary flare (not everyone experiences them though so don't worry if you've never had one) and with that, marked a change for the worse in my hands. Even though they were bad for the first twelve months, they really went downhill and were terrible for the whole of the second year. Out of nowhere, my left ankle also started flaring badly which was so swollen and oozy sometimes that I couldn't wear shoes. Then, as if a tap had suddenly been turned on, I started sweating profusely almost all the time. Because of these symptoms, which were only getting worse, my mental health also took a bashing. A typical day in the second year was definitely more normal though – eating three meals a day and trying to stick to some kind of routine. I was even able to go down to one shower a day.

The scratching was intense on my hands and ankle and even though I tried to ignore the near-constant irritation, sometimes it would get too much and I'd have to keep scratching until I felt like I'd almost reached my bones. Afterwards, there would be a split second of relief not to feel irritated before I was confronted with the damage I'd done. As my mum had long and incredibly strong nails, I used to plead with her to scratch me. She hated doing it, but I was desperate. Clothes were flung off during this period when the sweating started, which could be triggered by the smallest thing, or sometimes even nothing, and there were times where I'd wake up in the middle of the night drenched, and other occasions where I'd get slightly excited on the phone with friends and start sweating. It not only felt uncomfortable, but hurt, too, as it was like acid on skin where it was cracked and open. Mentally, after the first year where I was pretty positive that I'd get better, I really suffered – especially from month eighteen onwards – and started to question everything. I panicked that I'd never get better and thought that maybe I just had 'incurable' eczema and needed steroids and immunosuppressants for the rest of my life to function normally. There were days where I let myself go to a pretty dark place and as time passed, my conviction eroded, but I would never have used the drugs again which put me in this mess in the first place.

During the second year especially, I don't know what I would have done without reading, writing and talking to friends. I immersed myself in writing which proved to be the most extraordinary distraction and during the second year, I wrote one full length novel, a book of short stories, a novelette, and another short story which I then self-published on Amazon. Usually, if I wasn't writing, I was reading – or on really bad days when my hands were too swollen to write or pick up a book, I'd watch something lovely. I kept myself distracted where possible, but found the evenings hard – the time where I had to stop writing or take a break from reading. I'd see things for what they really were. I'd look at my hands which were so bad they felt like an out-of-body experience, and really let the doubt creep in. Fear, doubt and anxiety – always present and like a black cloud ready to storm. If I can offer you any real advice through this process it's to try and not let these feelings get the better of you – save yourself a lot of mental anguish and hold on to the belief that you will get better. My two-year TSW anniversary was bleak and I really thought on that day that I'd never get better ... but only two months later, I suddenly did. What a waste feeling like that was as now, when I look back, those days were precious – I was able to write; indulge in a passion I had found through this terrible process and also, without meaning to, changed as a person. I spent days thinking about my old life, pre-TSW, and all the terrible decisions, personally and professionally, I'd made. I realised where I had gone wrong, why I had such little belief in myself, where it stemmed from, and how I had got to this point. It really was transformative.

If you have a longer withdrawal like I did, remember that doubt and anxiety are just symptoms. Time passes, no matter how long, and one day this will be part of your past, like it is for me now, writing a book on a process that changed my life for the better.

MY TOP TIPS FOR GOING THROUGH TOPICAL STEROID WITHDRAWAL AND SOME REGRETS

I originally uploaded a video on this very subject when I set up my YouTube channel in 2015, but the problem with that video, along with others I posted around then, was that I had literally just got better and was understandably so excited that I didn't give myself any real time to think about what the hell I had just been through, and it's only since recovering that I have come to terms with what actually happened.

I am not going to recommend any dietary changes, moisturisers or drugs for the simple reason that we are all so different and what might help one person, might not necessarily be right for another. I believe with regard to food etc. that a balanced diet is best, but if you do 'cheat', the guilt you feel over having the offending food/drink item will be far more detrimental to your skin than anything you ate/drank in the first place. These are more universal tips that I believe could help most people going through TSW. I have also included a few things that I wish I had done during my own withdrawal.

• TIPS •

TAKE PHOTOS

I would highly recommend keeping a photo diary of your withdrawal because even though you might not feel like you are making any progress, photos will make you realise just how far you have come. Another reason is because when I got better and looked back over photos from my withdrawal, I couldn't believe how bad my skin was. I think your mind as a kindness sometimes blocks out certain tough memories and now those first few months of withdrawal are a blur. I am so grateful that I took photos. You don't need to do anything with them, but just knowing you have a record of what you went through, and survived, is empowering.

NO GUILT

Do not feel guilty about scratching your skin. I hear a lot of people berating themselves for doing just that.

Guys, it's impossible not to scratch sometimes. Where possible, try not to, but if you have to do it, just do it. This is a bit of a weird theory I have, but I believe you are actually *meant* to scratch. The body is trying to rid itself of the skin it doesn't want anymore, and the only way it can do that is for it to come off in flakes, or be scratched off. I am not advising you to rip your skin open with joie de vivre, I'm just telling you to give yourself a break from worrying about it so much.

DISTRACTIONS

Distract yourself as much as possible by concentrating on the things you love. For me, that was writing, reading Judith McNaught romance novels (I don't care, she is fabulous), rereading *Harry Potter*, watching *Jonathan Creek* reruns at one in the morning when I couldn't sleep – anything, just try to take your mind off what you are going through when you can.

KEEP COOL

Try to keep cool. I started withdrawal when the UK was in the middle of a heatwave and I can't tell you how much that added to my overall discomfort. In an attempt to make me feel more comfortable, my mum bought me an electric fan which made the world of difference. A lot of people also suggest using ice packs to kill the itch, but for those of us who don't have a freezer, what I found effective was filling a glass bottle with water, putting it in the fridge then rolling it over my skin. It was absolute bliss on irritated, hot skin and *sometimes* stopped me from scratching. Sometimes ...

DON'T OVERTHINK TSW

Don't overthink things, overanalyse what is happening to your skin or try to work out how long it will take to get better. Just try to trust the process and accept that time is the only true 'healer' of TSA.

MINDSET

Try to stay positive when you can. Knowing I wasn't using steroids anymore and was on a path to healing my 'eczema' really helped me stay focused.

YOU'RE HUMAN

On the days – months even – when everything feels too much, give in to it. Accept that you can't be positive every single moment of the day and just go with the motions of withdrawal.

COTTON PYJAMAS

Invest in some loose-fitting cotton pyjamas. For a long time, they were about the only thing my skin could tolerate. For UK sufferers, M&S sell reasonably-priced, but well-made, pyjamas that can withstand A LOT of abuse – from being washed constantly, covered in copious amounts of petroleum jelly, ooze, and all manner of fun stuff like that.

ACCEPTANCE

Where possible, try to accept any changes to your skin whether they are good or bad. This is something I struggled with until only recently and have had a few bouts of anxiety over small, innocuous rashes where I would panic that I was going to flare again. My rashes have never amounted to anything, but if you do end up flaring, remember that it won't last.

SHARE

Don't suffer in silence. When I was going through withdrawal, there wasn't much of an online community like there is now – all there appeared to be was a forum, but I found I couldn't go on there much as it depressed me. Now, there are the most wonderful Instagram and Facebook communities that I feel very lucky to be part of. Reach out and make some fabulous new friends who will understand everything you are going through, answer any questions or fears you might have and root for you every step of the way. Send me a comment or message via Instagram

(@carasnextchapter) and I'd love to follow your journey back to health.

• REGRETS •

DOUBT

I wish I had saved myself a fair few sleepless nights by always keeping the faith that I would get better. Doubt is a symptom of TSW that is not widely talked about which I find deeply sad as I think it can be one of the most destructive. Due to the nature of our condition we are fighting, on the whole, against a body of people we have been conditioned to listen to and trust implicitly: doctors. It is not their fault per se, and I have immense respect for their profession, but there must be a better understanding and education on the dangers of steroids to save others from having to go through a totally unnecessary process. Or, in the worst-case scenario where the person's skin is already addicted, having much-needed medical support for sufferers, because we are having to go through this traumatic period of our lives mostly on our own with only blind faith, and a handful of testimonials, to fall back on that we do actually get better.

Regardless of any doubt I experienced through my own withdrawal, there was no way I would EVER have gone back to using steroids again because I knew wholeheartedly they were not the answer and were only masking the real problem – not to mention how dangerous they are to use long-term. I did have some very dark times through withdrawal when I thought that maybe the doctors were right, I just had 'incurable' eczema. It didn't help that well over a year into withdrawal I had a long, stagnant phase where it was obvious I had improved, but was still suffering badly and certain areas were actually getting worse. There was also the fear that even though most of the swelling had gone down and I looked more like myself, I was still distorted by thick, irritated elephant skin and was scared that this was how I would look for the rest of my life and at times I'd torture myself by looking at old photos pre-TSW and couldn't imagine being that person again. Now, my skin is better than it EVER was before withdrawal – and that is without having to use anything on it. If I had ignored the doubt I felt and just accepted that I'd get there eventually, it would have made withdrawal SO much easier.

WRITE A DIARY

Oh my goodness, I can't tell you how much I regret not keeping a diary and logging everything that happened to me – or better yet, I wish I had started my blog from day one of TSW over four years ago. Now, I receive a lot of emails, messages and comments from others going through withdrawal asking me about various symptoms etc. that I experienced. Like I said earlier, I have forgotten so much of my own withdrawal and some periods are hazy. I am so grateful to my mum who, along with keeping a diary from the first month of withdrawal, dug up a lot of emails she sent to my aunt and uncle and a few close friends which read pretty much like diary entries that you will have probably read in this book by now.

MEDITATION

I strongly believe that stress was the main cause of my original eczema and now the multitude of studies that show just how much of a detrimental impact it can have in all areas speaks volumes. When I first got better, I introduced meditation into my daily routine and it made a huge difference to my appearance and general wellbeing. After a few months of meditating daily and absolutely loving it, life got in the way, and I found I was a lot more anxious without it. I'm not saying it 'heals' TSW, but I would like to have seen what impact it could have had on my withdrawal, at least mentally.

EXERCISE

I wish I had exercised a little more than I did instead of setting a new world record for sitting on the sofa. I think this is a little flippant of me to say though as in reality, I was in too much pain most of the time to even consider exercising, but looking back, I wish I had pushed through the pain as I really think it would have helped me.

MOISTURISER

I wish I hadn't used moisturiser from the beginning of withdrawal, especially petroleum jelly, which you will probably know by now after reading a whole chapter dedicated to the subject. After a lifetime of using moisturisers, I just assumed when I started withdrawal that I'd need them and at the time, most people's advice for dealing with TSW was to use petroleum jelly, which I did, but was very quickly sucked into this vicious cycle of being totally dependent on it to achieve a certain level of comfort and hating every minute. It was hellish, taking well over an hour to sink in – I have a memory from the first few months of withdrawal when the UK was in the middle of a heatwave and a daddy long-legs flew onto my shoulder and got stuck on my petroleum jelly-slicked skin … I did not enjoy that experience. It also wrecked my mum's washing machine and was an absolute nightmare to get out of my clothes. Use if you must, but with caution.

MAINTENANCE

I will never profess to having any kind of ritual or routine for TSW, and I don't believe that anything but time helps when it comes to symptoms of TSA, but as my diet/exercise/general routine is one of the most commonly asked questions I get, I thought I would share what I do in certain areas of my life to feel my best. I eat well for *me* and to look and feel good, but I am certainly not perfect, and I most definitely indulge on a regular basis. Again, this is not some miracle routine for TSW, and I am not a nutritionist or personal trainer – I'm just a woman trying to navigate her life and try, where possible, to do what's best.

~

• DIET •

I eat well, but I genuinely don't believe that diet has much of a bearing on TSW. We are essentially going through a drug withdrawal and time takes care of that *but* your body has been through a trauma and giving it food that will do it more harm than good is a disservice to yourself. It needs the right nutrients to repair and protect you. I can now eat and drink whatever I want (and trust me when I say that I've taken full advantage of that fact), but on the whole, I try where possible to give my body some love as a thank you for what it has helped me through over the years. The body and our ability to heal is an incredible thing.

When I say I eat well, that doesn't mean I am gluten-free, dairy-free, vegan or on any kind of restrictive diet. I eat a balanced diet which consists of a lot of oily fish, fruit, vegetables, grains, pulses, BREAD, DAIRY... I basically like real food. I have a lot of respect for people who can do such a restrictive diet – especially for ethical reasons – but as far as TSW is concerned, I don't believe it can 'heal'.

I found that during, and for about a year and a half after, withdrawal, I had a slight intolerance to strawberries, kiwi fruit and raw tomatoes and whenever I had any of them, my skin would tingle and feel irritated, especially on my lips. Now, even though I don't appear to have a problem with them, I still tread carefully, just in case.

Here is an example of what I eat in a day (during an average working week):

BREAKFAST

Porridge and blueberries made with semi-skimmed milk, and I don't use any added sweeteners like honey etc.

MID-MORNING SNACK

A handful of mixed nuts (unroasted/unsalted almonds, walnuts, brazils and cashews) with an apple.

LUNCH

Two hard-boiled eggs, a medium avocado, a banana and two to three small oranges. When I'm hungry, I'll add a flatbread or something else like salted popcorn, but mostly, I love how cleansing this is on its own.

I don't like snacking in the afternoon – just a personal preference (...unless someone has brought cupcakes or some other sugary concoction into the office and in that case, all bets are off).

DINNER

I tend to alternate between wholewheat pasta with passata, broccoli, spinach and mozzarella or tinned mackerel with broccoli, spinach and (microwavable...) brown rice. Whatever I eat, I almost always finish with plain probiotic yogurt.

Being a creature of habit, and having no time, has left me reaching for the same foods. At the weekend, I have much more variety but during the week, I actually really enjoy what I eat so don't feel the need to change it. I also stick to the hard-boiled eggs/avocados as it's really hard to find reasonably priced, but healthy lunches that don't have added sugar in them. Pretty much every day I will have spinach, broccoli, blueberries and avocados as I not only crave them, but believe their health benefits are nothing short of magical (maybe being a tad dramatic there, but you get my drift...).

I try to limit my sugar intake during the week, along with wheat (but the wheat's more of a gut issue) before all hell breaks loose at the weekend – although if I go out to dinner on a 'school night', I'll most certainly have what I want. I find that the quality of my skin when I don't have sugar is amazing – nothing to do with TSW symptoms and all to do with how I look and feel.

With regard to alcohol, I try to limit it where possible, but I do drink socially. I also tend to have wine and not spirits with sugary mixers, but that's only because I prefer them.

I think the beauty of going through something like TSW is that it makes you conscious of everything you put in your body and you get a strange sense of self-awareness. I try to eat intuitively and when my body craves chocolate, by god I'll give it chocolate. We have one life and you've got to find a happy medium otherwise you will look back and think, *I should have eaten that piece of cake.* Food is a pleasure and shouldn't be restricted.

At the weekend, my willpower is non-existent and my sugar content is high ... fabulous.

~

• EXERCISE •

This is not some kind of preventative measure for my skin, but on a daily basis, I exercise a lot in the form of walking. I walk to work, I walk during work, I walk at the weekends ... I just love it and probably end up walking for at least two hours a day. As time passes, I am realising the importance of physical activity and now, looking back, I wish I had done more whilst going through withdrawal.

~

• GENERAL DAILY RITUALS •

I rarely take long, hot showers – not that I consciously do it, more that I find I don't like to hang around as I've always got too much to do so it's a bonus that it's better for my skin. I also pat, not rub, my skin dry when I get out and never really take baths now. Whenever I am cleaning or washing up, I wear 100% cotton gloves under my rubber gloves which act as a barrier between not only the rubber, but the hot water, too. It is something I swear by and believe it makes a massive difference to my skin. I also try when I can to get at least seven to eight hours of sleep a night. It feels impossible to do that sometimes (try writing a book on TSW whilst working full-time …), but it's so worth it and I've found it makes a big difference to my skin when I get enough sleep, although I know that's so hard to do through TSW when your body has other ideas ...

• WINTER •

During the colder months, I will up my oily fish intake as a way of almost moisturising from within (probably a placebo effect though) and also monitor the central heating where possible as I believe this time of the year is when I'll see any kind of reaction on my skin. I wouldn't call it strong enough to be eczema – more a propensity for dry skin. Certainly nothing TSW-related.

• MEDITATION •

I do this for my general mental health and even though it sometimes gets pushed out of my day or forgotten, I try to do it as much as possible as I believe it is capable of extraordinary things.

• BE KIND TO YOURSELF •

Now, I tell myself that I am only human and that things will go wrong sometimes. The stress of any bad decision, meal or mistake you make is much more detrimental to your health than anything wrong or naughty you did in the first place.

• LIVE •

I live now – it's as simple as that. I can wear what I want and am not restricted by the colour or fabric of my clothes. I do what feels right for *me*. I walk till my feet hurt, I sweat like a normal person and feel the sun on my bare skin … I simply be. Being able to do all that is still a luxury and they are things which I know I will never take for granted ever again. That is the beauty of going through something like TSW – you treasure only the things that truly matter and *that* in itself is a gift not to be taken lightly.

1 8

MY CURRENT BEAUTY ROUTINE

his is probably going to be one of the shorter chapters in my book for the simple reason that I don't really have much of a routine. This couldn't be more different to before withdrawal where at one time I owned so many make-up and beauty products that someone asked whether I worked in the cosmetic industry (true story). When I went through TSW, the thought of any products on my skin was unbearable, and even now that I can use what I like, I don't want (or need) to. Pre-TSW, I wore thick foundation for two reasons: to cover the veins on my steroid-thinned skin that were especially obvious around my jawline, and because I simply had no confidence without it. TSW gave me a new perspective on everything – suddenly, I felt good in my own skin and wanted to be more natural, and so my routine changed accordingly. Now, I have a routine of sorts which works for <u>me</u>.

~

• BODY & SKIN •

I have a shower every morning and don't use anything on my skin apart from the *Dove Pure & Sensitive Hypoallergenic Beauty Cream Bar* only where I need it and while I'm in the shower, I'll wash my face using only warm water. I have found nothing gentler on my skin than Dove soap. I don't use any kind of face wash, and I am probably committing skin blasphemy here when I say this, but I don't use cleansers either as I really don't like the idea of stripping away all my natural oils. I am not a beauty professional, but after years of dry, barren skin, all my natural oils were hard to come by so the thought of mercilessly stripping them away from my poor, lonely face is madness. We all have different skin though, and I understand for some it's probably a necessity, but this is what feels right for me – for now at least.

I only wear eye make-up now which I take off with a bit of coconut oil (I love the *Lucy Bee Extra Virgin Coconut Oil*) on a cotton pad then use another pad to wipe off the excess before washing my face with warm water. Baths are a rarity, and I don't really hang around in the shower as I do believe that hot water dries out your skin. I try to pat myself dry when I get out of the shower before using my unperfumed Mum roll-on deodorant. Every second day, while I'm in the shower, I will shave my legs and under my arms using a *Gillette Venus razor* with a Sainsbury's own brand sensitive shave gel. On those days, I use the *Neutrogena Norwegian Formula Deep Moisture Body Lotion For Sensitive Skin* on my legs as I believe any kind of shave gel, no matter how gentle, does dry out the skin. Wonderfully, I now have no reaction to moisturiser and I absolutely LOVE the Neutrogena one. The day before shaving, I will dry body brush my legs, the tops of my arms and under my arms before getting in the shower to minimise ingrown hairs and reduce the likelihood of getting keratosis pilaris, which I occasionally suffer from, but much less when I stick to my dry body brushing routine. After my shower, I use the fabulous Neutrogena moisturiser on my legs again. I use the *Wilkinson Sword Quattro For Women Bikini Trimmer* for my bikini line (the electric shaver side and not the razor because I'm not a masochist). I don't use sun cream or any kind of sun protection which I know is a beauty crime, but I have yet to find one that doesn't make me rashy and after TSW, I find myself questioning if they are even worth it.

This is everything I do, but to be perfectly honest, the shaving/moisturiser routine is *occasionally* forgotten (… although don't tell anyone that).

• HAIR •

I wash my hair every four to five days or whenever I feel like it needs it. I have never had greasy hair so there is no real need to keep washing it – although after recovering from TSA, I definitely noticed that some of my natural oils returned to my scalp. On my naturally curly hair, I use a *Tangle Teezer* which is a game changer for getting rid of all knots without causing any damage before I wash it using the *Head & Shoulders Classic Clean Shampoo* followed by the *Pantene Pro-V Smooth & Sleek Conditioner*. I use a towelling hair turban – which is a MUST – then let it dry naturally. If I plan on straightening my hair, I will use the *TRESemmé Heat Defence Spray* beforehand then after straightening, run a tiny amount of coconut oil through my hair. If I leave my hair curly, I'll wait until it has dried before using the coconut oil.

A new discovery of mine is leaving coconut oil in my hair for as long as possible (which is usually about six to eight hours) before washing it as normal. It's very hard to find the time to do this whilst working full-time and having very busy weekends, but I try to do it where possible as it's made a MASSIVE difference to the condition of my hair.

• MAKE-UP •

I don't use any kind of primer, tinted-moisturiser, BB cream or foundation – I just use the brilliant *Collection Lasting Perfection Concealer* on the rare occasion that I get a spot or blemish, but that's it in terms of face make-up. I use a brow comb for my eyebrows and only take stray or errant hairs out as I like my eyebrows to be as natural as possible. To line my bottom lid, I use a taupe eye pencil from Rimmel and a black Rimmel Kohl liner for the top water line. I mostly wear a subtle cat eye most days using either a No7 pencil in 'Brown' or the *Rimmel Scandal Eyes Micro Liner* ... yes, you're right, I'm a big fan of Rimmel. I am besotted with the *Benefit Rollerlash Mascara* and now, I wouldn't dream of using anything else. On the days where I want to look more put together, I'll use some NYX eye shadow (two colours usually: one that is similar to my skin tone all over the lid then a mid-brown on the outer corners before blending). This all takes well under five minutes and is a far-cry from my pre-TSW days.

I am sure all beauty professionals are dismayed by my routine, but I love the freedom it offers me and besides,

I'd rather be living life than wasting time where I don't believe time is needed.

19

MY TOP TIPS FOR MEDITATION

*a*fter writing a whole chapter on anxiety in this book and talking extensively about how meditation can alleviate symptoms, I thought it might be a good idea to share some of the tips and tricks that have helped me meditate as I know from experience it can feel a little daunting knowing where to start.

I'm no expert, and I am sure I'm doing many things wrong, but these are the practices which have really helped me benefit from meditation and make it a thing of pleasure that I do almost every day. Meditation has really had such a positive impact on my mental health, and I hope these tips give you the push to try it for yourself.

GO SOMEWHERE QUIET

When you first start, you will probably find that every single sound is a distraction. Some noise is fine down the line when you know how to block it out, but while you are learning to clear your mind and be in the present moment, give yourself every chance possible by going somewhere quiet. Whether that means sitting in the bathroom with the door locked and the light off, or a quiet little nook in your home, find somewhere you know you won't be disturbed.

DARKNESS

Some meditations I have used say this isn't essential, but I find it really helps me to centre myself and be in the present moment when I am somewhere dark. When that isn't possible, or I'm meditating during the day, I wear a thick beanie hat which I bring down over my eyes that is not only comfortable, but blocks out any light. I have tried using a blindfold before, but didn't like the pressure around my eyes – the beanie is softer against your skin and less distracting. I also find that darkness tricks your mind into thinking you are somewhere peaceful as you tend to associate the dark with sleep and relaxation.

CREATE A PEACEFUL SPACE

Make a little peaceful area in your home where you go to for the sole purpose of meditating and when you get there, you know that is your space to be mindful. Surround yourself with the things that bring you joy and serenity – which brings me very nicely onto my next point ...

LIGHT A CANDLE

I suppose this is a pretty obvious point really, but I do believe that candles have the ability to transform any space and make it feel calm. After reading many worrying reports about the ingredients in a lot of candles out there, my mum invested in some that are 100% beeswax so completely natural and non-toxic. They have no scent, but what I find lovely about them is how they can bring so much warmth to any room, which is absolutely perfect for meditation.

GOOD POSTURE

I strongly suggest sitting up straight to meditate and not lying down. I've tried doing it like that before, but find when I'm lying down, I am distracted more easily ... or I simply doze off. I'd recommend sitting on a comfortable chair with your back straight and your hands placed gently in your lap. I find when I sit like this I am instantly centred and ready to meditate.

UNDERSTAND HOW IMPORTANT IT IS

I am still struggling to prioritise mediation and most days I go into it thinking I have more important things to do, but the last two years have shown me that I really need to keep striving for balance if I stand any chance of leading a life free from anxiety. What is the point of working hard but feeling so stressed and anxious that you are unable to reap the rewards?

REMEMBERING THAT THE TIME YOU TAKE TO MEDITATE IS ONLY A SMALL FRACTION OF YOUR DAY

Meditating for say fifteen minutes isn't exactly what you'd call a long period of time and anyone, regardless of their situation, more than likely has fifteen minutes they can spare. To put it in perspective, it's only a ninety-sixth of your day – that's it – and the things you think are more important will still get done.

GIVE IT TIME

I feel like this is the only advice I ever give these days, but I'm finding that time is usually the only answer I have. It's funny how sometimes the simplest of solutions are the hardest to implement. You are going to need to meditate for much longer than a few days to get any real benefits from it and I'd recommend trying it for at least four weeks to see what impact it can have on your mental health.

20

TAKING THE POSITIVE OUT OF THE NEGATIVE BUT WHY IT'S OK TO CRY SOMETIMES

One thing that had a massive impact on my withdrawal was staying positive. It wasn't intentional really and more how I was feeling at the time. That probably seems hard to believe seeing how much pain I was in, but in my mind, I was doing something that was nothing short of a miracle. I had dreamed for years of not using steroids, but had almost resigned myself to the fact that they'd always be a part of my life, so to suddenly have the chance of an existence without them and not have 'incurable' eczema any more was a risk I was more than willing to take. The moment I found out about Topical Steroid Addiction, I just knew wholeheartedly that *this* was what I had – it made total sense to me. Throughout withdrawal, I gravitated towards watching positive things and anything negative, I simply turned off or didn't read. I found Josh from the blog/YouTube channel 'Red Skin Recovery Diary' inspirational as he had one of the most laid back, positive outlooks on life that I'd ever come across and taught me that the bad times pass, and for both of us, they did.

Staying positive through TSW isn't something that is this constant shining light – it fades, it flickers and is so dark at times that you think the light has gone out, but through sheer force of will, it never did. Even during the later months of withdrawal where I really started to doubt whether I was doing was the right thing, I kept going, holding on to that deep-rooted belief that I would get better – and guess what? I *got* better.

For the most part, positivity is a choice. You are in an awful situation and only have two options on how to respond: you can either feel sad, angry and resentful towards the doctors or whoever prescribed you steroids in the first place, or you can find the positives in the now and build on them. There is nothing you can do about it and feeling negative isn't going to change things so why not be positive? Look on withdrawal as some much-needed time away and on the days where you would be going out but can't because of TSW, do something that makes you happy – whether it's binge watching a TV show on Netflix or rereading your favourite book. You could even be working towards something exciting for your future *after* TSW.

I was lucky enough not to have to work through withdrawal, but if you are in the position where you have to, or have family responsibilities etc., just think about the day where you will look back on all this and be amazed you were strong enough to persevere.

Having said all this, it would be near-on impossible to be positive all the time and I do actually believe there are moments where it is equally as important to let yourself really cry and give in to negative emotions. Like scratching, oozing and dry skin, bad times are inevitable and if it all becomes too much, just go with it. We are only human and aren't designed to be perfect – no one is – and being positive and happy the whole time is not viable.

Even though for the most part I chose to look on TSW as a positive experience, I was definitely not prepared for the incredible impact it would have on my life and how I felt about myself. Without meaning to, I made all these wonderful changes which I thought I'd share with you now.

I AM NOT USING STEROIDS ANYMORE

It goes without saying that not having to use a drug anymore, which was slowly damaging me internally as well as externally, is, in itself, something worth celebrating. Knowing I'm not dependant on anything was worth all the pain of withdrawal. I can't tell you how trapped I felt by my addiction and couldn't go anywhere for more than a few hours without a tube of steroid cream to hand. Before TSW, I felt like a prisoner in my own skin and for that reason alone, I would gladly go through it all over again if it meant I got to be free, like I am now ... but please don't make me go through that again :)

FREEDOM

Continuing on from my last point, I have had to spend most of my life thinking about my skin in one way or another. In the past, there have been cupboards bursting with bath preparations, creams, ointments, immunosuppressants and topical steroids and I could never stay over at a friend's house or go away on holiday without what felt like a whole pharmacy in my suitcase. Now, I don't need anything to maintain my skin and could go anywhere I like with only a small tub of coconut oil to remove my eye make-up. I can just step out of the shower without thinking of approximately eight thousand things I need to put on my skin in order to function like a normal person.

This seems silly, but I am sure that anyone with eczema or TSA will understand when I say that for many years I would look longingly at people who could, for example, get out of the sea or a swimming pool and simply be and not have to rush to slather themselves in their trusty moisturisers. I don't have to worry about things like that anymore and it's life-changing. The freedom of not having think about my skin is a gift I would never have been given without going through TSW and for that alone, my gratitude is immense.

I AM GRATEFUL FOR MY HEALTH

You realise just how extraordinary the human body is and how it is constantly fighting to protect you. All I wanted to do when I was going through withdrawal was wear a nice top and walk down the street. Sounds absurd I know, but that simple act I had taken for granted for so long now became a precious commodity I wanted more than anything in the world. Now, being able to feel the sun on my skin is something truly magical and I know that no matter what happens, I will always value what it means to be well.

TIME TO THINK

I was lucky enough to not have to work through withdrawal which meant I could hide away from the world and, as a result, was given the most incredible opportunity to think – think about my life and all the choices I had made which had led to my life-altering present. Sometimes those thoughts were more painful than the symptoms of TSW for I realised some damning home truths which I could pretty much pinpoint back to a very specific period in my life and how that experience shaped me. Now, even though I might not be completely over it, I at least understand why.

SELF-BELIEF

This is still a work in progress as I have had to rebuild something that was completely and utterly broken for a very long time, but as time passes, I am slowly finding pieces of my self-belief and putting them back together again. For many years, I wanted to sing – very much – but never had the belief in myself to really go for it. I was terrified of rejection and being told that I simply wasn't good enough because in my head, that was exactly how I already thought of myself. I felt like I didn't deserve the best, both personally and professionally, which resulted in jobs I hated and men that weren't good enough. Now, I fight for what I want and if something isn't right or I know I deserve better, I walk away.

WRITING

I will try and put this across without being corny or cliché, but I simply found my passion in life because of

TSW. I'd spent a long time thinking about writing, but for many years, I was too scared – of what, I don't know. I remember the autumn before withdrawal, I had an idea for a novel which made me so excited that I jotted down all these ideas and characters for it, but well over seven months later, those ideas only gathered dust … until five days before withdrawal when suddenly, I was just writing, and it was wonderful. During TSW, I wrote two full-length novels, a book of short stories, a novelette, and another short story – not to mention all the invaluable time in which I simply practiced the very act of it. After TSW, I was armed with all these incredible tools and had in my possession actual books that I had written. Nearly five years later, that passion is still well and truly alive and only burning brighter. All this is not to say that I'm any good at it – more that I love it and won't stop for anything in the world … told you my self-belief was still a work in progress.

R-E-S-P-E-C-T

This is something I've only just come to realise, but now, I have a newfound respect for myself and will walk away from situations (and people) that I know aren't right or good for me. I found this out when I actively started dating again after a *very* long break. Before TSW, I would go along with situations that I knew weren't good for me, but as I didn't have enough respect for myself to leave, I persevered. Now, I will put up with very little and if I know a person isn't right or they do something that hurts me, I will simply leave, and even though it might be hard (or sometimes a little heart-breaking) to do so, I will do what I believe to be right, and if that means I am single for all eternity while surrounded by twelve cats, then so be it. Life is too short to be in situations which make you essentially unhappy, and even though some decisions are scary at the time, long-term, you know they are the best thing you could ever do for yourself and almost always mean that something better is just around the corner. We live in a self-deprecating society where we fear loving ourselves, but that is the most selfless thing you can do.

APPRECIATING THE THINGS THAT MATTER

When you go through something as life-altering as TSW, you come to realise who your friends are and what really matters in life. Material things are suddenly irrelevant. We only have one life, so let's use it wisely.

THE IMPORTANCE OF KINDNESS

When you come to understand the things that matter in life, you also realise just how important it is to be kind. Kindness is one of the simplest but most powerful things you can do for yourself and the people around you. You must find balance though as some will take advantage of that kindness and attempt to walk all over you. I'm still striving for a happy medium, but nevertheless, it has already made such a positive impact on my life.

SLAYING SOME OTHER MONSTERS

At the top of every New Year's resolutions list I ever made was to stop using steroids. A close runner up which went even further back than steroids was to finally find a way of overcoming Trichotillomania and Dermatillomania; two compulsions which have had such a detrimental impact on my life, trapping me just as much as the drugs my skin relied on. I developed both Trichotillomania and Dermatillomania at a time where I was deeply unhappy and for about sixteen years, they played a massive part in my life ... until the day where I decided they weren't going to be there anymore, which I would never have been able to say if I hadn't gone through Topical Steroid Withdrawal. TSW taught me that I was stronger than I thought and if I could get through that, I could do anything ... and so I did. On the 7th October 2016, I vowed that I would find a way to eliminate those two final demons from my life and over a period of seven weeks, I managed to do just that. It certainly wasn't easy and there have been times I've given in, but I can safely say that they no longer play a part in my life.

Even though TSW is undeniably tough, you will find there are times where you have a choice how to feel about your situation ... so what will it be?

21

THREE SMALL WORDS

This is a little story about what it means for me to not give up on something, come out the other side and find my passion along the way.

❧

Through a lack of self-belief and a rather severe fear of failure, I spent most of my teenage and young adult life running in the opposite direction from any opportunity that came my way and in turn, missed out on things that I now can't look back on without feeling a sharp pang of regret. I had absolutely no confidence in myself and what I was capable of and chose to work hard in the wrong areas through fear that if I put my heart and soul into the things I truly wanted, but failed, I would have wasted time and been absolutely devastated. It was easier in a way thinking about what *could* have been than trying and possibly failing. As a result, I spent many years quitting and giving up on my dreams. For a long time, I wanted to be a singer, so I set up a MySpace music page then, as it grew, I started a YouTube channel until over time, I had gained a small but ever-growing fan base and was even getting the odd singing job off the back of it without even trying ... but what did I do? I gave up because I was scared. I loved it so much that I quit rather than really try and to this day, I can't think too much about singing and what might have been. Who knows, I might have ended up failing, but I'll never know and now, I don't want to. Around 2012, I set up a fashion/beauty YouTube channel and blog, but when I started getting an audience, what did I do? I gave up. A year later, I set up another blog ... and what did I do? You guessed it.

I would say in the months leading up to withdrawal, everything was coming to a bit of a head. I had a great social life and loved my friends and family, but personally, I was going nowhere. I remember Monday 20th May 2013 vividly as it was a turning point in my life. I was in the middle of a shift at a job that had absolutely no prospects and on this particular day, I was asked to work in a different area where I was made to feel absolutely useless by other staff members. At one point, I pretended to go to the bathroom, but instead, I ran to a deserted corridor, hid behind a pillar, and cried my eyes out. I remember thinking to myself, *what the hell was I doing with my life?* I had spent *years* wasting time in these jobs through fear and where had that thinking got me? I had a job I hated and was crying in an empty corridor. It was at that moment that I knew I needed to change my life completely. For a few months, my skin had been worrying me – I'd started having a lot of trouble with my eyes and rashes were appearing over my body that no amount of topical steroids were clearing. Even worse was the fact that my skin was thinning badly and I had developed some kind of allergy to the sun. Around this time, I went to the doctors feeling absolutely desperate, but their only advice to me was to use stronger steroids. Even then I knew that was just a slippery slope, but I didn't know what to do.

Over the following few weeks, I did a lot of thinking about my life and on the 1st June 2013, after years of wanting to write, but being too scared to, I finally took the plunge and, in that moment, fell head over heels in love with it. Five days later, on 6th June 2013, I found out about TSW, had my lightbulb moment and changed my life. I always get a little choked up when I think back to the moment where I realised I didn't have 'incurable' eczema, but Topical Steroid Addiction – it was the most sure I've been about anything in my life and in a way, the answer almost seemed so obvious that I couldn't believe I hadn't thought of it in the first place. I remember experiencing such a concentrated form of relief and knew with all my heart that Topical Steroid Withdrawal was the right thing to do, and even in those two plus years where I doubted the process and questioned if I really did just have eczema, I never gave up. For the first time in my life I gritted my teeth and held on for dear life to something I totally believed in and after just over two years, the storm finally cleared and my 'incurable' eczema was gone, leaving in its wake better skin than I'd ever had in my life.

TSW was the first thing I ever did where I just kept going – ignoring those that didn't think TSA existed and fighting my own doubts along the way. The process taught me three words which I will spend the rest of my life being eternally grateful for: Don't. Give. Up. TSW taught me that if you keep pushing – keep fighting for what you believe in – you will get there eventually. For years, I thought I'd have to use steroids for the rest of my life to treat my 'incurable' eczema – I'd almost resigned myself to the fact and was paying the price with thinning skin and photosensitivity, but in the end, I went against what I was told and did what I believed to be right, and won.

Writing through withdrawal became my passion and in those twenty-six/twenty-seven months, I did things I never thought I was capable of, so not only was it nice to come out of TSW with all these actual books I had written, but the knowledge I had found the thing I wanted to do for the rest of my life.

To anyone going through withdrawal, find something that brings you joy and gives you a sense of purpose. Hold onto it tightly and let it guide you through the storm.

22

TSW TEARS ON VALENTINE'S DAY

I originally posted this on my blog on Valentine's Day 2017,
and as it went down so well, I thought I'd share it with you
all here, too.

~

If my memory serves me correctly, I cried three times during Topical Steroid Withdrawal. Don't get me wrong, I cried *many* times through that period, and I'm still recovering from watching the film *War Horse*, but I'm talking more specifically about TSW being the cause, and in that case, I can only think of three occasions where I really let the tears fall.

The first time I cried I think I was well over a month into withdrawal – more like two – so we are talking about a time where I was full body flaring. On that particular day, I also experienced nerve pain and the feeling of bugs crawling all over my skin – plus, I was just so tired from the sheer lack of sleep and completely confused and scared that I burst into tears of futility. The second time I cried was a few months later and was once more down to a mix of tiredness, pain and fear. I even remember where I was sitting when I cried. Strange the details you remember sometimes.

The third time was on Valentine's Day two years ago. For a while up to that point I'd not been doing so well. My hands seemed to want to outdo themselves on how bad they could get, I was SO uncomfortable and I had really started to let doubt in. No matter how positive your approach to withdrawal is, chances are you are going to feel a little scared/doubtful/worried from time to time.

Well anyway, as the day wore on, all I seemed to see online were girls excited to get ready to go out that night – they were getting their hair done, putting make-up on and wearing fabulous clothes. There wasn't a specific image or person that sent me over the edge, but all of a sudden I was crying – really crying. I wept for the life that had been taken away from me. I wept for not being able to do the same as those girls. I wept for not knowing when (or *if*) I'd get better. I wept hard. I hasten to add this had pretty much nothing to do with the man/date itself – more knowing that I couldn't do anything I wanted to. At this point I couldn't even leave the house or, let's be real, change out of my pyjamas. Ultimately, I just wanted to be a woman again and didn't care whether it was going out with a group of girlfriends for the night or just having the choice, but I think that was definitely the lowest day of my withdrawal. When I then add that only a mere six months later my skin suddenly transformed, I think it says a lot. Even now, I am learning to be more open-minded about anything that comes my way as even the smallest rash can still be the catalyst to a breakdown ... but after all these experiences and years of having to second guess what my skin is going to do, I am trying to retain some faith that everything is going to be OK – and so far, it is. I sit here with skin I never dreamed I'd have in my life – no steroids, no immunosuppressants ... the list goes on.

This year I'm most likely watching *Gilmore Girls* (my new favourite thing) then *Sex and the City* with my mum, who I live with, which might not sound like a twenty-something woman (nearing thirty – I'm in denial) living life to the full, but it's *my* choice. The reason quite simply is that I have not met a man I want to date and since going through TSW, my standards have pretty much skyrocketed. I feel like I deserve more now and know what I want. In reality, that means I am holding out for an exact replica of Tom Selleck. If you have read my Trichotillomania diary, you'll know I've been single for a long time and I can most definitely already hear the pitter-patter of tiny feet (I'm talking about the cats, naturally) waiting for me to welcome them into their new home as I more than likely enter my thirties single ... en route to the convent.

If you are going to be indoors tonight in your pyjamas because you are not well enough, or, you are better like me, but choosing to stay indoors, let's make a pact regardless that the person we say we love this year is ourselves. The love of Yourself is by far the hardest partner you will ever have to woo. So, from one friend to another, I want you to look in the mirror and say, 'I love you' today because you are SO worth it.

23

SOME TSW-RELATED THOUGHTS

Another chapter I originally posted on my blog back in May 2017. It's small and sweet, but I thought it might be worth including in here, too.

~

Since I have started writing a book all about my experience of going through TSW, it has forced me to think about a lot of things I've tried to forget, but seeing as I am very close to reaching four years of Topical Steroid Withdrawal, I thought I'd share some thoughts that have been on my mind lately.

One thing in particular that has amazed me is how TSW, which was such a huge part of my life for so long, now feels like some kind of dream and it is only in the moments where I get a rash and my anxiety goes into overdrive, or I really force myself to think about the experience, do I remember what I have been through – the scratching, the sleepless nights, the oozing ... all of it. Now, it all feels like it happened to someone else ... but how can something that *was* my life now feel like it never existed?

I suppose it's a pretty fortunate question to find myself pondering, but still, I'm stunned how easily I've been able to forget just how hard those two plus years were. I suppose pain is like that though, isn't it? I remember years ago when I'd just had two wisdom teeth out and got an infection, the pain was unlike anything I'd ever experienced in my life, and as I sat in A&E feeling like I would never be comfortable again, I made a solemn vow that I would never take my health for granted ... but of course, I forgot all about that and carried on with my life – or perhaps you have a particularly bad period pain that is severe enough to make you never want to have children ... until you feel better and get all broody. Pain is temporary and to anyone reading this, there will be a time where you'll forget all this discomfort and pain you are going through and be able to appreciate the present. Don't get me wrong though, I am still healing from TSW mentally, but physically, I think I've moved on and soon, I know my mind will follow.

Over time, as my hands have gone from strength to strength, I find myself looking at them almost in awe, completely baffled that the skin has healed the way it has. I have said this before, but looking at my hands at certain points during the second year of withdrawal especially was as if I was looking at someone else's hands. Now, I can't for the life of me remember exactly how it felt to not be able to move them properly or the pain of scratching them until they bled.

Even though I have forgotten so much of the pain I went through during TSW, one thing is for certain: I will NEVER take anything for granted again – whether it's my health, just feeling comfortable or knowing what a pleasure it is to do something as simple as feeling the sun on my skin. The small moments are precious to me, and I will do everything in my power to hold onto them.

I don't know if there was much point in posting this, but I feel like it has been bubbling up inside me for a while now and I hope it at least helped someone out there remember that one day, TSW will be a part of their past, too.

24

A LETTER TO MY TSW SELF

Another chapter taken from my blog and written back in August 2016 ...

~

*N*ext Wednesday will mark exactly a year since I got better. Incredibly, just a few days before things suddenly changed for me, my future was hazy. I remember when I passed my second year TSW anniversary last June I felt, to be perfectly honest, a little cheated – I had made massive progress, but was stuck in this long, stagnant phase and was still really struggling with my hands and left ankle, to the point that it significantly limited what I could do each day. In celebration of my upcoming landmark, I thought I'd write a letter to the me of a year ago in the hope it can help some of you who are fed up and losing faith in TSW.

Dear tired & lost Cara of July/August 2015,

You have been dealing with this isolating, debilitating condition for over two years now. Most of the medical profession don't believe what you are going through is real with one doctor saying there's a quicker way to recover if you start his treatment plan involving topical steroids again, the people who you know and love are wondering if you are doing the right thing and even you (though you will never actually admit it) have questioned if whether going through this was just one giant mistake. You can't even wash your own hair or wear shoes much because your ankle is swollen and on top of that, you sweat like a waterfall if you so much as sneeze. You look at old pictures of yourself and ask why you never appreciated what you took for granted and are constantly thinking, will I ever look like that again?

Darling Cara (you may be shocked at the term of endearment you have given to yourself, but in the next year you will realise you need to love yourself), in a matter of days something miraculous will happen: you are going to get better. You are going to wake up one morning, look in the mirror and see someone new. You are going to be beyond ecstatic in the months to come, but also terrified that it is all just an illusion and in turn, be constantly preparing for the worst at any moment. It'll take you a while, but there will come a time when you realise nothing is guaranteed and you will start to force yourself to live for every single moment and appreciate this new skin you have worked so hard for. Go feel the sun on your skin (maybe wear a hat though, because you end up collecting a few more freckles than you should), eat the damn chocolate (because it won't make a blind bit of difference) and revel in all the mistakes you will make as this time next year, you'll realise just how much you have learnt about yourself. You are going to change a lot, and it's going to feel uncomfortable for a long time, but wonderfully you will learn that without going through Topical Steroid Withdrawal, you would never have been able to become the person you are today.

(And please scratch that desperately itchy skin if you need to.)

Love,
Cara of the 14th August 2016 x

JUST IN CASE

Like the previous few chapters, this has also been taken from
my blog and was originally written in December 2016.

~

On Instagram, I follow a lot of people who are in the throes of withdrawal and over time I have noticed the same worries and fears come up that hang over our condition like a pall until we are not only fighting the truly awful physical symptoms of withdrawal, but also battling the demons inside our head that are constantly telling us we are doing the wrong thing. With that being said, I thought I would put together a few reminders for anyone who is struggling right now in the hope that it acts as a little tonic to help keep the monsters in your head at bay.

I suppose in a way I am writing this to the me of a

few years ago in the midst of withdrawal – the girl who was scared at times that maybe she did just have eczema and all the doctors and dermatologists were right; the only answer was to use stronger steroids and immunosuppressants for life to have any semblance of normality. I know this path can feel like the wrong one, but in reality, it is the best thing you will ever do for you and your skin, and I believe that overcoming the symptoms in your mind is the real challenge of TSW ... not convinced? Well just take a moment to think about what would happen if you took away all those doubts and fears ...

There is no such thing as backwards, only forwards, and even though it may not feel like it, every day that passes brings you one day closer to recovery.

You WILL get better and are not the anomaly who just has eczema. If you are on this journey, you are on it because you have TSA. The decision to go through something like TSW is not normally made because of some arbitrary whim you had – if you are on this journey, you are on it for a pretty concrete reason.

Remember why you started TSW – the desperation you felt followed by the relief when you realised you had found the answer you had been waiting for. In the moments where you feel like giving up and just want to go back to using steroids, think about what compelled you to stop using them in the first place – why did you stop?

Anxiety, doubt and fear are the <u>worst</u> symptoms of TSW.

Recovery is not linear. There will be ups and downs and most will not gradually get better. There might be a long period of calm followed by a flare that takes your breath away, or you might be in what feels like a perpetual flare, but whatever you do, don't be discouraged because at any given time you are always one day closer to getting better.

Elephant skin goes. Just like the oedema, weeping skin and bone-deep itching, elephant skin is a <u>symptom</u> of TSW and only temporary.

Feeling guilty for scratching is like feeling guilty for breathing. Scratching is inevitable.

This process takes time, and lots of it. Time is the only true 'healer' of TSW.

Give yourself a pat on the back – you're doing the best you can.

Never feel guilty. Period.

Do not compare your withdrawal to another person's as it will only lead to disappointment and anxiety. How long it takes to recover differs from person to person.

Eat the damn cake if you want to.

You are not alone.

Don't suffer in silence as we are all fighting in one way or another.

THE ONE TRUE HEALER OF TSW

*A*s I am getting older, I am realising that time is the only thing which truly heals all wounds, regardless of whether they are physical or emotional ones. You split up with someone and time comes to the rescue to repair all the wreckage invisible to the naked eye. You break your leg and time is there once more to slowly put you back together again. The same can be said for TSW and now I find that time is the only real advice I can offer because even though we are all so different, in this one thing, we are bound by the fact that it *will* take time, and lots of it.

The problem we now face is that we live in a society where we all want a quick fix, and that is essentially what steroids do – they mask problems, leaving them bubbling under the surface waiting for the moment we stop using them to pounce again. Now, we have pills for everything which is a wonderful thing, but as a result, we have become lazy – scared of a bit of discomfort when in reality we should be taking a little longer to find an answer which could save us a lifetime of pain.

The two most commonly asked questions I get now are about my diet and how long I think it will take them to 'heal' – some have said things like, *I've been going through withdrawal for two months and I'm still not better* ... There are some who 'heal' within a year and I could not be happier for them, but for most people, that won't be the case as we are not simply dealing with a skin condition here, we are trying to repair sometimes decades worth of damage, internally and externally, and expecting your body and skin to just bounce back from that and recover quickly is madness. It's odd, but my mum, friends and family all thought I'd get better within a matter of months – I never did. I knew this was going to take time and because I believed in the process more than anything, I kept going, gritted my teeth and tried to accept that I would get there eventually. That didn't stop the fear and anxiety from creeping in, especially in the second year, with that small voice in the back of my head telling me I would never get better and just had 'incurable' eczema, but I let time do its magic and after twenty-six/twenty-seven months, I came out the other side, grateful I stuck with it.

I want to say again that Topical Steroid Addiction is so much *more* than a skin condition – it's an all-encompassing monster, and you can throw celery juice at your system eight thousand times a day, wear only the finest Egyptian cotton and bathe in the purest apple cider vinegar, but the only thing that will make you better is time. Let your body do what it's meant to and by all means, eat well and do what you can to look after yourself, but don't expect it to be some magical answer. You'll get better when you're meant to so save yourself a lot of unnecessary pain overanalysing and stressing about the *when* and just appreciate that it *will* happen … eventually.

27

MY VIEWS ON ...

Sometimes, this whole experience feels like it has turned me into a dermatologist or something as every day, I am asked for my opinion on things that are shrouded in uncertainty. I am not a medical professional and have never professed to be – I am simply a woman who has overcome a rather horrific condition. With that being said, I *have* spent over twenty-five years of my life having to deal with my skin in one way or another and while my opinions aren't validated by a degree, I believe it does offer me a *degree* of understanding – another perspective. This is my issue with the way eczema is treated by most of the western world – just smother symptoms and pretend they don't exist rather than dealing with the root cause. Twenty-five years' worth of doctor's appointments and pretty much all they have done is reached for that tome-like book to search for yet another steroid or immunosuppressant to throw at my condition. Doctors are wonderful, no doubt about it, I am simply more concerned by the way they are being educated on how to 'manage' (I think you might have gathered that I hate that word by now) eczema. I have some views that could be considered controversial, but to me, they are born from common sense. These opinions are not here to convert you to my way of thinking – they are merely answering the questions I get on a daily basis. I am not asking you to agree with me and I am *definitely* not asking you to change my mind because I won't. Everything that surrounds TSW is very close to my heart and over time that has made me passionate about the things I truly believe in, so read this with caution ... and an open mind.

• DIET & TSW •

I think the most commonly asked question I get is to do with my diet. *What diet did you follow to heal? Did/do you take any supplements ...?* the list is endless. Even though I do not believe that diet can 'heal' Topical Steroid Addiction, I think it is vitally important in a broader sense. Your body is going though, or has been through, a trauma, and your skin – more like your whole system – is doing everything it can to get better, so you need to fuel it right to help it along and give it some much-needed love. I have always eaten relatively well. I love real food and eat a variety of fruits and vegetables. If I ever get a scab, it heals pretty fast, and I believe *that* (along with genetics) is down to my diet.

TSW is essentially a drug withdrawal and while I believe that you do get better regardless, your body needs the right nutrients to support recovery ... so in a broader sense, I suppose you could say that a good diet both during and after TSW is essential and even though it might not 'heal' symptoms, you are helping yourself in the long term. Don't see food as a quick fix, see it as an investment in your future. Most importantly, I would like to state that when I say 'eat healthily', I don't mean you have to be a vegan or do something drastic like that – I'm talking REAL, less processed, whole foods. Now, I try to limit my sugar intake where possible as I do believe it is an irritant, and while taking out sugar isn't going to magically heal symptoms, I do think a generally bad diet can exacerbate any underlying issues. This could all be a placebo, but it's what I believe.

When I first recovered from TSW, I was so desperate to stay well that I overhauled my already pretty healthy diet and took refined sugar and things like honey etc. out for about three to four months and the difference in the quality of my skin was quite staggering. I also try to avoid things like bread and pasta sauces that contain added sugar as it feels a little redundant – if I want a chocolate bar, the game is up,

I'm having sugar, but I certainly don't want it in savoury food.

Post-TSW, you find that you are hyper-aware of everything you put in your body and what feels right for you, so start listening to what it is saying and surprise yourself when you realise you can actually hear it telling you.

• IMMUNOSUPPRESSANTS •

In my (non-medical) opinion, immunosuppressants are just as bad as steroids and when you throw in the fact that they are also used to prevent the body rejecting transplanted organs and tissues it begs the question, *why* should they ever be used to treat skin conditions in the first place?

Back when I was reliant on steroids, I would use immunosuppressants occasionally in lieu of the steroids as I was desperate for an alternative and knew how much damage they were doing to me. The immunosuppressants would keep my skin just as clear, which should be warning enough not to use them, and the side effects for the ones I used were simply terrifying. Protopic in my opinion should be banned. When I was first prescribed it in my teens, none of the links to cancer were talked about and I was told to apply it liberally. I hated it. I hated the smell of it when it had sunk into my skin, the burning when you came into contact with water, having to completely hide away in the sun and the red flush you got if you even thought about drinking alcohol. I used it a few times on and off over the years, but had to stop as I developed an alarming number of freckles, even when I'd been careful enough not to go in the sun. I had photos taken of them at the hospital and I know that stuff caused me so much untold damage. Now of course, the possible link to cancer is widely known and talked about, but it scares me how easily it was prescribed back then. Why are cancerous drugs a better alternative to finding out what's actually causing eczema in the first place? We don't need more immunosuppressants out there, we need a better understanding of a condition a lot of us have had to deal with for many years.

I think it is important for me to state again that this is not a medical opinion, it is simply one woman's experience. I feel it is also vital to say that this is not a criticism of anyone currently using them. I have so much love and respect for our community and would hate to feel like I'm judging anyone, but it's got to the point where I feel like I've got to say something. I believe immunosuppressants are just as bad as steroids and when we talk about going through withdrawal, it should be from ALL of the drugs that suppress our system in one way or another. I feel I can say that as someone who has not only used them, but been burnt by them (quite literally in my case …).

As Topical Steroid Addiction can take such a long time to recover from, I understand how some people might want to turn to an immunosuppressant as a means of finding some relief – trust me, I get it, I just don't see how it's any different to using steroids. I was lucky as I didn't have to work through withdrawal and could just concentrate on getting better, and I genuinely don't know how some are able to go to jobs and school or look after children etc. as I found it hard enough as a single adult female with no real responsibilities.

If you are currently looking into treatments to alleviate symptoms of TSA, all I ask is that you give the option of immunosuppressants a lot of thought. Do your research and work out what would be best for YOU in the long run.

• SCRATCHING •

I am probably in the minority here, but I believe scratching to be an important part of withdrawal. I am not giving you licence to rip your skin open, I am simply saying that I think scratching is the body's way of naturally removing the skin it doesn't need any more. I believe it is the same with oozing – your body is doing everything it can to get better and as there are so many chemicals in our system to get rid of and damage to repair, symptoms are going to be intense.

All I'm really trying to say here is that when you can, don't scratch, but if you've got to, *whatever* you do, do NOT feel guilty for doing something that would be impossible to resist. Not scratching through TSW belongs in a land where pigs fly …

I have many other opinions that I would have liked to include in this chapter, but they would've inevitably had a rather negative impact on the book, and I want this to be more about my journey and not focused on debating topics which are already hotly contested. Through TSW, you've got to learn what works for YOU and make up your own mind about what you believe to be the right thing to do.

28

SO YOU'RE IN IT FOR THE
LONG HAUL

*D*ue to the nature of our condition, and a startling lack of information, there is no magic answer or crystal ball telling us just how long TSW will take. For some, it's a handful of months – for others, years, and I unfortunately fell into the latter category. Yes, it's demoralising when you look at other people recovering faster, or better, than you and you're not able to understand why, but the beauty of life is that we are all different, with different genetic makeup, and because of that alone, you must NEVER compare your withdrawal to another person's as it will inevitably lead to some kind of breakdown. For twenty-six months and eleven days I was in withdrawal. Most people around me thought I'd be better in six months, and I certainly don't think anyone was expecting over two years ... apart from me. I mean, I definitely questioned the process, as you well know –

I felt like giving up many times and had these moments of pure madness where I'd think how easy it would be to just use steroids again – but I knew this wasn't going to be a walk in the park and I most definitely knew I'd need a substantial amount of time to recover. I used steroids cumulatively for well over ten years – I only say it was ten as that is what I can safely guarantee, but it's probably a lot more.

Topical Steroid Withdrawal is not as simple as having a little scratch and it all being over. Through this process, we not only have to repair our broken skin, but our adrenal glands, sweat glands, nerves … the list is endless. Topical Steroid Addiction isn't a skin condition, it is a total body trauma, and expecting the process to be quick is crazy. We are essentially having to rebuild our bodies from 'scratch' so need to appreciate the gravity of what we are asking of it. Our bodies have sometimes had to withstand years of drug abuse, so to then get it working again on its own, without the need for something it has relied on for so long, is a massive undertaking. For over twenty-six months I watched my skin do things – terrible things – I didn't know it was capable of. I then watched in fascination as it turned into the best skin of my life.

Regardless of all that, what I wasn't prepared for was the non-linear nature of the recovery process. Mine was all over the place and as certain parts of my body got better, others decided to get worse. Mentally, that takes its toll and as a result, irrationality can take over even the most rational of minds. Anxiety is clever in that way – it can mess with your head to such an extent that it has the ability to make you question everything you once believed in.

I was very ill for twenty-six months. I didn't have periods of calm where I could live – even a little – and physically, life was hellish. I couldn't really go out for long periods of time without feeling either so uncomfortable that I wanted to rip all my clothes off because I couldn't bear them on my skin or having to endure the acid-like burning. My body had to start again. My sweat glands were completely confused and my blood vessels had to find a way of waking up after years of enforced sleep – not to mention my skin, which had to remember how to fend for itself. Mentally, I needed the same amount of time – if not longer – to recover.

Drugs can be a wonderful thing, but they do make our bodies lazy and now I have recovered, I am absolutely fascinated by what the body, without the need of artificial help, is capable of – how it can heal, protect us …

When I said I was writing this book, I was asked to share my thoughts on those who were still suffering at three, four years in. I do not understand why some of us take such a short time to get better then for others, the journey is so long … so all you can do really is embrace the unpredictability of life and accept that we are all different. You are not someone else's withdrawal and you are most certainly not alone. You went into this process believing that you would get better – remember how excited you felt, that wonderful moment when you realised there was indeed an answer. Hold onto that thought and remember this is only temporary.

Even in those desperate moments where steroids and immunosuppressants look like such an escape – an easy way out – think about a time in the future when they will inevitably stop working and make you feel desperate again. They are not an answer; they only prolong the inevitable and put you in this mess in the first place. We have been thrown into a situation we should never have go through. This is not just a skin condition we are recovering from, this is something which affects us in every way imaginable – mentally, physically, internally, externally …

Think of it as one massive jigsaw puzzle – it will take time to put all the pieces back together again, but one day, you will be whole.

29

CELEBRATING THE MILESTONES

*J*f you know me or have followed my story for long enough, then you'll know I love a good milestone. I have spent years using them as fresh starts, a slate being wiped completely clean, and while I am realising that living that way can do more harm than good – to hold so much store by what is essentially another day – I do believe that it is *vitally* important in the case of TSW. We need something to hold onto, to work towards. A way of grounding ourselves; a reminder that time does indeed pass and with it, comes ever-better skin.

On my one-year TSW anniversary, I marked the occasion by buying a pretty lifestyle book that I used as inspiration for when I'd get better and be able to live again. It brought me a lot of pleasure and if you are not well enough, like I was at the time (hello anniversary flare!), buy yourself a small token – it doesn't have to be expensive – which will keep you going and act as a sort of goal. Something you will be able to use or do when you get better.

My two-year anniversary was a very dark day and the last thing I felt like doing was celebrating another year passing. I was consumed by doubt and fear that I'd never get better and started to wonder if all I had was 'incurable' eczema and my only choice was to use steroids and immunosuppressants for the rest of my life. On that day, two years in, everything looked so bleak, and I remember thinking of all the time I'd thrown away on something I thought I believed in. It was then, only two months later, that I made a sudden and full recovery … so that is what I'd call a rather wasted opportunity for a celebration.

In a bid to make up for the previous year, my third anniversary was nothing short of wonderful. The weekend before, my mum (who was just as big a part of my withdrawal as I was) and I had a fabulous day out together. We went to a restaurant I had wanted to go to for ages (the Ivy Brasserie in Kensington) then had a tourist day in London, eating macaroons in Ladurée and window shopping in Harrods. My mum also bought me a beautiful necklace; three silver intertwined circles to represent the three years of withdrawal. I wear it every day and in the moments where something stressful happens, the necklace reminds me of everything I have been through and that the bad times don't last. On my actual anniversary, I started writing in *A Page a Day – My Five Year Diary* as a way of marking it as a fresh start – a new phase in my life – which I have continued writing in every single day since. Life is this crazy, ever-changing rollercoaster and we've got to appreciate and celebrate the highs to get us through the lows.

Year four wasn't really marked in a big way due to the fact I was moving back to London in a few weeks' time and was busy with that, but as I knew I was working towards a life I was SO excited to live, that anniversary, although still marked in a small way, was more a happy passing of time, which is *exactly* what I wanted.

I have something rather big planned for my fifth anniversary … but I'll keep that a secret for now. It's somewhere I've always wanted to go and will truly mark the end of TSW for me. I say *end* as a way of mentally closing the door on that chapter of my life. My experience of going through TSW will always be with me, but only the good which has come out of it, and that in itself is something to celebrate.

30

SOME FAQS

Some of these frequently asked questions have been taken from my blog, whilst others have been added to cover everything else I have been asked over the last few years.

∼

How long did you use topical steroids for?
I used topical steroids cumulatively for WELL over ten years. This is only a rough estimate, and I am sure it is much longer than that, but it's the only figure I can be totally sure of. I used a course of oral steroids in my teens then mostly milder steroid creams like Eumovate and hydrocortisone twice a day throughout most of my 'addiction'. I also used Betnovate and other stronger steroid creams, but that was in the earlier stages of my dependency.

Have you ever taken oral steroids?
Yes. I took one course of what I believe was Prednisone in my teens and part of me thinks that was when I developed TSA.

How long did it take for you to 'heal'?
I don't think I can ever bring myself to use the word 'heal', but I will say that my skin suddenly changed for the better after twenty-six/twenty-seven months of withdrawal and since then, I've only experienced mild rashes and two isolated flares on my hands which lasted a matter of days and not months like during withdrawal.

Did you find that when you got better, it was sudden or gradual?
For me, it was the case of one day looking at my skin and realising I was better. Really. It's been well over two years since that happened and I still don't think it has actually sunk in.

Why do you think you got better when you did?
As time goes on, the more I think that you get better
when you're meant to and my withdrawal had simply
run its course. I have said many times that I think a
healthy diet is important BUT I believe you get better
regardless. I also think that things like steroid usage,
age, climate etc. play a part … but could someone just
research this already and give us some peace of mind.

**Do you think you can withdraw from topical
steroids slowly to ease symptoms of withdrawal?**
Honestly, no. I think you just have to do it cold turkey.
I think it differs depending on what steroids you used
though and might not be safe to do so (e.g. oral
steroids) so do a lot of research before embarking on
this and *please* seek medical advice. www.ITSAN.org is
the mothership for all things Topical Steroid
Withdrawal so I would definitely recommend visiting
the site before you do anything else. I should also
mention that over the years I tried weaning myself
down to the lowest amount of steroid cream possible,
but it was only when I stopped using them completely
that my 'eczema' would come back severely.

Did you have any 'breaks' during withdrawal?
In a word, no. I had slightly calmer phases followed by bad flares, but no breaks where I could actually live my life. It was pretty debilitating for me throughout the entire two years of withdrawal.

Were you able to work while going through TSW?
No, not at all. I tried working for the first three weeks of withdrawal but after that, it was actually my mum who stopped me from going and said she would support me. I was pretty much housebound for over two years.

Did you experience oozing?
Oh my *goodness* yes. I oozed from my face, neck, chest, arms, back, left ankle and hands. Luckily, it only lasted on the whole for the first three months with more isolated oozing on my hands and left ankle later on. It's a draining part of the process (quite literally) and when it stopped, the relief was immense.

Did you suffer from oedema?

Yes, very badly in my arms to begin with, along with my face, neck and back. It slowly went down during the first six to twelve months of withdrawal.

Did you experience any hair loss during TSW?

Unfortunately, yes. I lost a lot of hair especially around my hairline and eyebrows, but it all grew back.

Did you sweat excessively through withdrawal?

I certainly did – more like I was a human waterfall. It was in the second year of withdrawal when the sweating started and out of all the symptoms, this was something I found extremely hard to deal with. Without moving much at all, there were times where I would be covered in sweat. I would wake up drenched in it, and if I got excited in any way – even just talking to a friend on the phone – I would sweat profusely. A lot of people say it's a sign that the body is healing and now, looking back, I would tend to agree. My sweating is completely back to normal now and has been since I recovered over two years ago.

Did you suffer from insomnia?
I didn't sleep much for the first year of withdrawal and during the first six months especially, I barely got more than two hours in one go. This is extremely tough to deal with as you spend your days exhausted and desperate to sleep, but can't when you have the chance to.

Did/do you suffer with anxiety?
Absolutely, and there are many chapters in this book which prove how much of an impact it had on my life both during and *after* withdrawal.

Do you suffer from asthma?
No.

What did you use to combat the elephant skin?
The best remedy for elephant skin is time. It goes, just trust the process.

Do you think there is a link between periods and flaring?

Honestly for me, there hasn't appeared to be any link. One day I might start to see a pattern forming, but the rashes I get tend to be sporadic.

Now that you are better, do you still get itchy?

Not really. On the very rare occasions that I ever do get itchy, it's just a mild irritation that I can ignore and definitely not that bone-deep itch you experience while going through withdrawal – more like a feather gently tickling my skin.

What do you eat?

I eat a balanced diet which I talk about in more detail throughout the book, including chapter twenty-one: 'MAINTENANCE' where I even break down what I eat during a typical workday.

~

Do you believe in a healthy diet?
I talk about my views on diet and TSW over many
chapters in this book (including chapter thirty-one:
'MY VIEWS ON').

~

Did/do you take any supplements?
No.

~

Have you tried apple cider vinegar or Epsom salt?
Nope, never wanted to – although I have heard
absolutely wonderful things about both.

~

**Have you ever used Protopic? If so, what are your
views on it?**
I have used Protopic in the past and my views are, to be
blunt, extremely negative. I talk about this in more
detail in chapter thirty-one: 'MY VIEWS ON ...' under
the section on immunosuppressants.

Did you use any drugs to ease symptoms?
Bar the odd antihistamine, I used absolutely no drugs to alleviate symptoms, my thoughts being that I was withdrawing from one drug and didn't want to replace it with something else – I almost wanted to flush out my entire system. I also found that antihistamines weren't worth it so in the end, I didn't even bother taking them. I know there are others who take various drugs to ease symptoms during withdrawal, which I totally understand, but not having anything felt right for me at the time and through this process you've got to do what's best for YOU.

How did you tackle the loss of movement and flaking whilst doing Moisturiser Withdrawal (MW)?
I think because I did Moisturiser Withdrawal so slowly, I was somewhat able to control the flaking and movement. I talk about my whole MW experience in chapter thirteen. I did have a hard time especially through the colder months though where my skin was extremely dry and cracked so I decided when it got really bad to use moisturiser again, but that didn't work out very well which I also talk about in more detail later in the chapter.

∾

What skincare/make-up do you use?
I share my entire beauty routine in a chapter rather appropriately called, 'MY CURRENT BEAUTY ROUTINE'.

∾

Why do you never say that you have healed when you obviously have?
I have a few reasons why I don't (and will never) use the word to describe my journey. For the most part, and this probably sounds a little strange, but I find it to be a little flat. TSW is multifaceted and recovery is never linear or final. It takes time after the physical symptoms have abated for the mental ones to catch up. There will be rashes and panic attacks and terrible memories. I feel comfortable in saying that I have recovered – healing is like it never existed and because of that, I don't want to 'heal' as that would mean I wouldn't have learned all these valuable lessons about me and my life from the experience of going through TSW. It changed me for the better and I never want to forget that. I also believe that the moment I use it to describe my journey, I am only tempting fate and remember many people using the word before flaring again – almost as if they jinxed themselves. Say and do whatever you like – this is only my opinion. We all

have to find ourselves to a certain degree through this process and discover what works for us.

What do you have to say to anyone who is struggling and debating whether to use steroids again?
When I say that Topical Steroid Withdrawal was one of the best things I have ever done, I mean it wholeheartedly. Before withdrawal, all my life in one way or another I had to think about my skin. I was told countless times that eczema was 'incurable' and that the only treatments available to me were steroids or immunosuppressants. On Thursday 6th June 2013, when I found out about TSW, it felt like a weight had been lifted off my shoulders. The answer made total sense to me and even though it took a long time to get to the stage I am now, it was never really an option to use steroids again as they offered no real solution to the actual problem.

To anyone suffering at the moment, ask yourself if steroids are the answer. If you broke down and used them again, think about what would happen in the future. Where do you go when the strongest ones stop working? This process is immensely tough but SO worth it. Try to stay realistic about how long the process will take and NEVER say by X date I will be 'healed' – just take every day as it comes and <u>always</u> remember that you WILL get better in the end.

RESOURCES AND IMPORTANT
WEBSITES

I have said it before, but I look on our community as one big extended family. When I started TSW back in 2013, there were very few people documenting their journeys but now there are so many blogs and videos about TSA and TSW that it's hard to know where to start. Because of that, I thought I would highlight the people, blogs and websites that have helped me through my own withdrawal and some I have discovered in the two years since recovering.

~

ITSAN
(www.ITSAN.org)
I think most people reading this book will already know about ITSAN, but I couldn't really start this chapter without talking about them first. ITSAN

stands for the International Topical Steroid Addiction Network and is pretty much the mothership of our condition. Set up in 2009 by fellow TSA sufferer, Kelly Palace, it aims to spread awareness and educate those who have, or think they might have, Topical Steroid Addiction. Naturally, this is a must-visit website as it provides so much information on our condition.

≈

Dr. Marvin Rapaport
(*www.red-skin-syndrome.com*)
Not his website so much (not that it isn't brilliant) and more the man himself that I wanted to discuss. In a nutshell, Dr. Rapaport is a US-based dermatologist who believes Topical Steroid Addiction exists. With over thirty-five years' experience, he talks about our condition with so much common sense and passion. I remember watching interviews with him on YouTube that I turned to when I needed a bit of reassurance. He also offers consultations either in person or remotely which can be arranged through his website.

≈

Dr. Fukaya
(*www.mototsugufukaya.blogspot.co.uk*)
Again, another doctor who wants to spread awareness for our condition. Based in Japan, his blog is

immensely helpful and has so much information on it for anyone going through TSW, or wishing to learn more.

~

Jake & Libby's blog
(*www.eczemahealing.blogspot.co.uk*)
This was the first blog I read which convinced me that Topical Steroid Withdrawal was the right thing to do – it also helped my mum for the same reason. To see what he went through, then how he recovered, kept me going. The blog is written by his girlfriend (now fiancée) who logged his highs and lows and looked after him. A <u>must</u> visit for anyone going through, or thinking of going through, withdrawal.

~

Josh's blog with links to his YouTube channel
(*www.redskinrecoverydiary.blogspot.com*)
Josh is an Australian guy who went through TSW and one of my all-time favourites. His laid-back attitude and positivity was exactly what I needed and made me want to be the same.

~

The Bond's founding principles

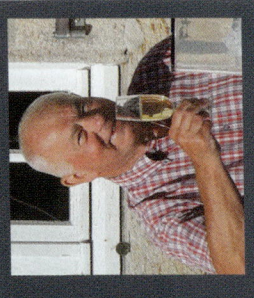

Holidays, food, wine...

Living it up at HPB's
Manoir du Hilguy

page 10

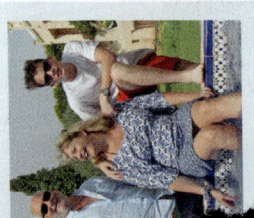

The insider guide to the
Holiday Property Bond

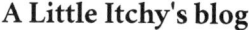

A Little Itchy's blog
(*www.alittleitchy.blogspot.com*)
This blog hasn't got much content, but it's one hell of a transformation story. When she posted a picture of her 'healed' hands, I kid you not, I saved the page as a bookmark on my laptop and would stare at her porcelain skin for long periods of time to keep going. Even though there isn't much on the blog, it is still definitely worth checking out.

Juliana's blog
(*www.antisteroid.wordpress.com*)
Juliana is the true embodiment of a skin warrior. She's had a very long, tough withdrawal and her blog has helped me so much throughout my own journey.

Nina Sloan's YouTube channel
(*www.youtube.com/channel/UCbbb3z6ItXZoge-vGt0d91A*)
I had the pleasure of meeting Nina when we filmed the documentary on TSA (*Preventable: Protecting Our Largest Organ*) together. While I was going through TSW, her videos, which she uploaded on YouTube,

were an inspiration to me and document each stage of her relatively short withdrawal (eight months).

… And lastly, here are two new discoveries:

Briana Banos
(www.youtube.com/channel/ UCGul7qzTlVJ6fOfHKV2ao8A)
I first came across her YouTube channel just after recovering in September 2015 and her videos on TSW are simply brilliant. Funny, informative and poignant in equal measure, I couldn't recommend them enough to anyone going through, or thinking of going through, Topical Steroid Withdrawal. This year (2017), she shared that she would be making a documentary on our condition called *Preventable: Protecting Our Largest Organ* which I had the pleasure of being part of this summer. To find out more about the documentary, visit www.preventabledoc.com.

Nina's YouTube channel
(www.youtube.com/channel/ UCrQMqNdY201OxxOUstxqmqw)
A very raw channel showing just how tough TSW can be. Nina was incredibly brave and filmed when she was

at her most vulnerable which will make you cry and want to reach out and give her a big hug.

I also want to quickly mention the names of the four TSW Facebook groups I am part of:

- Topical Steroid Withdrawal-Red Skin Syndrome Support Group.
- Eczema & Topical Steroid Withdrawal for WOMEN-Healing Through Positivity.
- ITSAN Topical Steroid Withdrawal Syndrome Support Group.
- TSW London Network.

The Facebook groups are something I wish I'd known about when I was suffering as they are wonderful. Not only are they fantastic for support, but there is always someone there to answer any questions you might have on TSW within minutes. It's also fascinating seeing how quickly all the groups are growing and I am curious how many members they will have as time goes by.

There were a few other resources I turned to whilst going through Topical Steroid Withdrawal, but they have since been taken down. The reasons are usually to do with the author's need to move on from it all, which I totally understand, but it does make it hard on those who are left behind. When I started withdrawal, there was very little out there in the way of help and support, but now there is so much and as time passes, it is only getting bigger. In a way, it's a double-edged sword: knowing that as others find out about TSA, there will be more people suffering temporarily, but on the flipside, it also means more will find an answer to their 'incurable' eczema.

32

IT'S THE SMALL THINGS

*A*s my book comes to an end, I thought it might be nice to begin another story: yours. Grab a notebook, or even use an app on your phone, to write one positive or thing you are grateful for today – whether it's an empowering quote or even something as small as saying you made it through another day (which at times during TSW feels nothing short of a miracle). At the end of withdrawal, you can then look back over your entries to see how far you have come. Even if you don't feel like doing this right now, try it anyway to see what happens. Who knows, you might even surprise yourself when you realise that by focusing only on the positive, it has an impact on the way you see everything.

33

AN UPDATE

Written on Saturday 27th July 2019

This week, after reading through my book for the first time since publishing it in December 2017, I thought the time had come to write some kind of follow-up – an update of sorts – because a lot can happen in a year and a half, and I think it's only right, due to the nature of the book and my particular skin story, for there to be total transparency.

This probably sounds a little strange, but I was almost scared to read through it again because, quite simply, I'd forgotten what I had written. Apart from jotting down a few rough chapters at the beginning of 2017, the main body of the book was done over seven rather intense weeks leading up to publication. When I finally read through it again this week, I got a bit of a shock, because all I could think was, *did that really happen to me?* Suddenly, all these suppressed (appropriate word under the circumstances) memories came flooding back, and I'm not going to lie to you, it was tough. Of course, I'm so happy I wrote it, and to have such an important piece of my life in one place, but it's quite hard to be suddenly transported back to that time. Since writing the book, a lot has changed, but some things have stayed the same.

I have just passed my six-year TSW anniversary, and in keeping with my love of celebrating the milestones, Mum and I put on some pretty outfits and had a rather wonderful afternoon tea together at Sketch in London (the place with the Instagrammable toilets …). It was amazing, and whilst I'll always feel something every 6th June, as time passes, I forget a little bit more of what I went through for over two years because essentially TSW is no longer a part of my life.

A lot of people ask me how I am able to be so present in the TSW community and answer questions on a daily basis about such a harrowing time, and I do it for two reasons:

1. More than anything, I understand the importance of being there – showing that there is light at the end of the tunnel. The mind through TSW is a fragile thing, and to have something solid to hold onto and keep you going through the darkness is <u>vital</u>. I needed that so badly through my own

withdrawal at a time where there wasn't much of it available.

2. Quite simply, over time, I have found a way to disconnect – like there is a chip in my head which enables me to go into autopilot because now it's as if someone else went through withdrawal and not me. I talked in the book about how fickle humans can be when it comes to pain, and it's true. Our mind can be so tough on us, but sometimes, it can be kind, too, and soften the sharp edges of whatever trauma we went through – comfort us, tell us it wasn't so bad. This week, when my mum and I read through certain sections of the book, we turned towards each other in shock, suddenly remembering just how hard TSW was, because she was just as much a part of my withdrawal as I was. We might be the ones in physical pain, but our loved ones are in pain, too, just in a totally different way, so be kind to them, always.

You're probably wondering how my skin is now, and quite simply, I don't remember the last time I had a rash. Really. Over time, the skin on my face has gone from strength to strength and it's only really my hands that have had any kind of reaction; getting slightly chapped when the temperature suddenly takes a nosedive, but that's like most people in the world really, regardless of whether they have a skin condition or not. Even my flatmate who has no issues said last winter that he struggled to wash his hands once as they were so sore from the cold. After withdrawal, we aren't little china dolls with perfect skin – we have skin that will react to the elements because we are human.

In the book, I discussed some symptoms that I was still experiencing after withdrawal that are now non-existent, including:

- Nerve pain and the feeling of thousands of bugs crawling over my body. To be honest, I forgot all about this until I read through the book this week. Thank GOD I wrote it all down because it appears I have no memory ...
- Hot/burning skin. Absolutely nothing like this has happened since publication.
- I mentioned that I used to get dry lips if I had cold/flu symptoms or ate too much sugar – not anymore, and when you hear about my diet in the last few months, you will know I have certainly not shied away from the sweet stuff ...

The only thing I still suffer from is anxiety, but it is a different beast entirely to what it once was and is now absolutely nothing to do with TSW. I mean, it might be the case that withdrawal made me anxious and it just decided to stick around because Pandora's box had already been opened and there was no way of closing it again, but regardless, I no longer have a fear of flaring and instead, it is now triggered by a lack of sleep and pushing myself too hard. I have social anxiety, too, born from the isolation of TSW, but I know that will go in time, and in a way, I prefer who I am now. I may have been louder before TSW, but all that noise was only silencing how I really felt about myself, and it wasn't good. If I'm being completely honest, my anxiety is actually worse now, but I know I don't help myself. If you suffer with it, too, then you will probably agree that there are warning signs you tend to ignore till it's too late and you are stuck on the hamster wheel and can't get off, with your thoughts spiralling dangerously out of control. I have also been told it's likely I have anxiety-induced IBS, too, as now, when I'm anxious, I bloat like a goat who has eaten bread. After a couple of really bad bouts of anxiety this year, I had to take a step back, forced myself to not do anything but my full-time job and waited till it calmed down again. Meditation helps, along with not eating as much sugar which seems to exacerbate it – but have I actually done either of those things? Of course not.

Oh sugar ... Sugar and I have been in a very turbulent and passionate love affair over the last five or six months, and I can safely say my diet has never been so bad. Ready for my excuse, and it's a good one ... recently, I realised that since I was a little girl with eczema, I have had to think about everything I ate, as if some omnipresent being was always there, ready to judge my food choices and how it might affect my skin. But I think it dawned on me at some point this year that whatever I ate didn't appear to affect my skin, and so for the first time in over thirty years I have had TOTAL FOOD FREEDOM, and I've gone feral. My addiction to sugar has got to the point where I've started calling it my boyfriend. Make of that what you will and is probably a story for another day ...

I still love healthy food and couldn't live without it, but I have certainly padded out my diet with far more junk than I ever have before, and whilst my skin has been fine, I feel crappy. Now, sometimes I think I'm infallible because I feel so strong after withdrawal, but it's taken these recent bouts of anxiety, teamed with a poor diet, to remind me I am human and can only push myself so far. I am attempting to eat better again because I want to, and that's pretty lovely – not doing something because of my skin, but for me. How novel.

Diet is such a controversial subject within our community and as far I'm concerned, I don't believe there is much of a link between food and flaring. I think a lot of people forget whilst going through TSW that it is essentially a DRUG WITHDRAWAL and not a regular skin condition. I still believe that certain foods can exacerbate symptoms, but not cure them, and I have yet to see anyone prove me wrong, although I am over the moon for those who think a radical diet change has helped them. We are one community who all want the same thing: skin freedom, and so we should stick together and support each other, no matter what route we take to get there.

My beauty routine is pretty much the same as it was before, apart from finding the hair care brand Kérastase, which has been a game changer for my Hagrid-prone hair – although I still use the Head & Shoulders shampoo because it is just brilliant. I also wear sunscreen now. I said in the book that in the past I had reacted to every one I had tried – that was until I found Sunsense. Sunsense is an Australian brand that a wonderful blog reader recommended to me last summer. Now, I use their Ultra 500 SPF50+ Sun Screen which is lightweight and so gentle, and since I've used it, I haven't had any kind of reaction. I wear it every day, even in winter, and I'll never be without it. Although with that being said, part of me still feels it's wrong using one at all … but as a freckled redhead, I can't take the risk that my (probably crazy) theory is wrong.

On the whole, my views have not changed – give it time and don't give up. Time. That is all it boils down to really – and I mean *real* time, not a handful of months. TSW is a marathon, not a sprint, so try not to listen to the voices telling you you'll never get better and to just give up. When something gets uncomfortable, no matter how much we want it, we all have a tendency to want to run – forget about the reason which led us to take a particular path in the first place. I have to tell myself that all the time with writing now. I am working full-time whilst also trying to make writing my career, but I'm so tired. I get anxious as a result of pushing myself too hard and there have been mornings where I've already been writing for a few hours then have to force myself out of the door to begin a whole day at work. It's lucky as I really like my day job, but that doesn't mean it's been easy, balancing the two, and sometimes that familiar voice I heard all the time during withdrawal will come back and ask me, *is it all worth it?* But because of what I went through, now, I grit my teeth and keep going because not giving up through TSW turned out to be the best decision I ever made and I ended up with skin I had been desperate for my entire life.

Something that has upset me since recovering is doctors' disinterest in TSW. There have been times where I've seen the doctor for something unrelated to my skin, then after asking if a particular treatment they have prescribed has any kind of steroid in it and I start to tell them about TSW, I see their eyes glaze over. They just aren't interested. I totally understand how hard their job is, and I have so much respect for all that they do, but it does upset me that they aren't ever just a little bit curious to hear me out – and that kind of response is why we have a problem in the first place. It is imperative that there is a better understanding and education on the dangers of these drugs so no one has to suffer as we have. Although saying that, the opinion within the medical community as a whole seems to be changing for the better. Awareness is spreading, and on Instagram alone there are now twenty-five THOUSAND photos on the hashtag #topicalsteroidwithdrawal. It's wonderful, as it means word is getting out there, but it also means that more people are having to go through something they should never have to go through in the first place. Maybe one day people will know the dangers of these drugs and never become addicted, but just like TSW, it's going to take time.

Something very exciting that I wanted to talk about is the documentary on Topical Steroid Addiction, *Preventable: Protecting our Largest Organ*, which was released this March and is absolutely wonderful. So far, it has had over 37,000 views on YouTube, with the National Eczema Association even putting a link to the documentary on their website. Our condition is finally being taken seriously, and, even better, now, we have not only one, but TWO documentaries on TSW, with another one in the works which I was lucky enough to be a part of last year.

I wanted to end this chapter by saying thank you. When I wrote the book, I had no idea what would happen after I published it. This was always a passion project for me – a way to finally say goodbye to TSW and close a door on that 'chapter' of my life. I thought at least my mum would buy a copy, but what I wasn't expecting was the extraordinary response from the skin community who made the whole experience so incredibly special. I have been stunned by the reviews and posts about the book, the kind messages ... from the bottom of my heart, thank you.

And so all that leaves me to say is goodbye to an old foe – or friend, you decide.

TSW, you changed me. I grew, I made mistakes, I learned from them, I fought, and I won.

Love,
Cara x

ACKNOWLEDGEMENTS

I think I could only start this off by thanking the internet for guiding me to Topical Steroid Addiction. There will not be a day where I don't feel grateful for the answer I had been waiting a very long time to find.

To ITSAN, Dr. Rapaport, Dr. Fukaya, and the countless blogs and videos which kept me going through withdrawal. *Thank* you.

To my TSW family, for your courage, love and support which inspires me every single day.

To my friends and family, for showing me the most extraordinary kindness and love throughout the entirety of my withdrawal (and beyond). I will never be able to thank you enough.

To Cari, for opening my eyes to the world of Judith McNaught romance novels and as a result, leaving me disillusioned by men in the real world. Thank you for being such a wonderful friend.

To Hugo, for your friendship throughout withdrawal ... and your advice ;)

To Johan, for our two-hour-plus phone calls which kept me sane (I still haven't got a clue what we talked about), but most importantly, my eternal love and thanks for sending me DIEUX DU STADE, the French Rugby Team's Nude Calendar 2014.

And finally, to my mum, Elaine. I could write another book just about what you did for me through withdrawal, but instead, I will simply say, from the bottom of my heart, thank you. I love you to the moon and back.

ABOUT THE AUTHOR

Cara started writing in 2013 after falling in love with it whilst housebound from the iatrogenic condition, Topical Steroid Addiction, which she has since made a full recovery from. She is now an advocate for the relatively unknown condition which affects thousands of people around the world. Cara also has a popular blog about her skin journey which can be found here: www.tswcara.blogspot.com

In December 2017, she released the book, *Curing my Incurable Eczema*, about her battle with Topical Steroid Addiction, which reached the top five in the dermatology book charts on Amazon. In April 2019, she released the short story, *Just Julia*, based on her own experience of living with eczema. Her first collection of short stories, *Thirty-Minute Tales*, was released in September 2021.

Between late 2014 and early 2018, Cara wrote the women's fiction series, *Weighting to Live*, which was republished in 2022. Around the same time, she also published the standalone short story, *Knock Down Ginger*, inspired by her experience of being bullied because of the colour of her hair.

Sign up to the mailing list to receive your monthly newsletter and author updates here:
www.cararward.com/join

For more information, visit:
www.cararward.com &
www.authorcaraward.blogspot.com

instagram.com/carasnextchapter
goodreads.com/authorcaraward

OTHER BOOKS BY
CARA WARD

JUST JULIA: A SHORT STORY ABOUT ECZEMA

'I just need one day of not being in this body.'

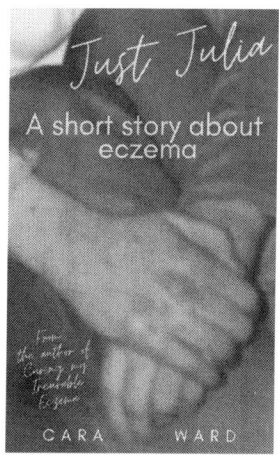

Julia Ross is a twenty-something woman (barely) living with eczema.

Julia Ross has been told not to scratch.

Julia Ross has been told to use coconut oil.

Julia Ross has been told it's never going to get better.

Julia Ross has come to the end.

Can Julia Ross reclaim her identity from her skin or has she finally given up?

Based on the author's own experience with eczema, this short story hits home on exactly what it's like to live with a condition most people believe is only skin deep.

Available to download for FREE on Amazon, Apple Books, Kobo, Nook, Google Play Books, and many more

Printed in Dunstable, United Kingdom